"Propagated from the an 'urban jungle' into an ir ing the less obvious applic tice. Sweetlife Flora now teaches others how to integrate plants into their lives and motivates veterans to look forward to their next plant therapy session for it has innumerable health benefits."

-Christina Connelly, CD, CRSP, CRST, CEO
Chief Facilitator of Kompass Health Associates Inc.
www.soldier2self.com

"Brilliantly written and inspiring for horticultural therapists and those who know the value of people and plant relationships. Kristin has bridged the gap between negativity and despair to hope and healing, bringing new purpose and life for those who experience trauma and depression."

-Mitchell L. Hewson, HTM, LT, RAHP | Administrator
Horticultural Therapy in Practice
www.horticultureastherapy.com

"An unabashed account of one's journey prior to and living with a traumatic brain injury. Kristin embodies the ethos of 'Never Give Up' and offers an enlightening story of self-discovery and self-improvement. A testament to the healing power of horticulture."

-Greg Bucci

The Story of How My
Indoor Garden Saved My Life

PROPAGATED FROM THE ASHES

Chantale,
Thank you so much
for supporting me! I'm
so pleased that we've met.
I hope I can help with
your transition to
civilian life!

♡. Kristin

KRISTIN TOPPING
Sweetlife Flora

Published in Canada for Global Distribution by Golden Brick Road Publishing House Inc. Printed in North America.

ISBN: 9781988736600

Author: info@sweetlifeflora.ca

Media: hello@gbrph.ca

Book orders: orders@gbrph.ca

Contents

Prologue

A Library of Impressions

This isn't a sad story, quite the opposite, it is a record of my journey and recognition of how my indoor plant collection saved me from the depths of depression. Over the course of my adult life, I suffered multiple minor traumatic brain injuries (mTBIs). The impact of the repeated concussive injuries meant that I became more susceptible to further head injury. In December 2016, I was the victim of a fluke, random accident involving a roller coaster at a theme park. My life changed unimaginably in the blink of an eye. I, like so many others who have sustained a traumatic brain injury, have suffered physically and most markedly, mentally. The person I am today looks nothing like the person I was in 2016. This is a story of personal loss, mourning, and most importantly, recovery.

My life is divided into three distinct parts: before the accident, immediately post-accident, and life after the accident. I'm sure many people who experience trauma can identify with this multi-reality situation. When I'm asked to recall a certain part of my history, it is like opening a different book from a totally separate section of the library. This book is very dusty; the print is faint and hard to read. Sometimes the pages are stuck together and won't come apart, no matter how hard I try; other pages have been completely torn from the binding; and sometimes, the print from one page has bled onto the next. That's how it works with traumatic brain injuries, you're left with fragments of a story here, blended memories there, convoluted impressions of a past that may or may not have happened exactly the way you remember it—this is where my story of renewal begins.

My recovery is an ongoing process, particularly as I redefine my definition of recovery. I no longer define "complete recovery" to mean I need to be the person I was before, I know that isn't possible, nor do I even want to be that person anymore. The concept of who I am and the expectations I have for myself have been refined. I am proud of who I have become, and I look forward to the future. None of this would have been possible without the collective support of my loving family, an open-minded primary care physician, a very patient physiotherapist, several occupational therapists, multiple mental health professionals, and a slew of neuro-specialists. But most of all, I attribute the recovery of my mental health, and many aspects of my physical health, to a self-care regime that focuses on the care, maintenance, and collection of houseplants. I refer to this practice as *mindful horticulture*. It is a self-care practice for anyone, not just those who have been affected by injury or trauma. I will lead you through the background and tenets behind this practice, giving you tips and tricks for how you can accommodate it into your lifestyle. I would not be where I am today without my urban jungle, it quite literally, saved my life.

If you are inspired to take notes or jot down thoughts while reading, please do; a notes section has been included in this recovery memoir near the end of the book for you to use. You can also contact me if you have further questions or feedback, see Appendix 4 for my contact information.

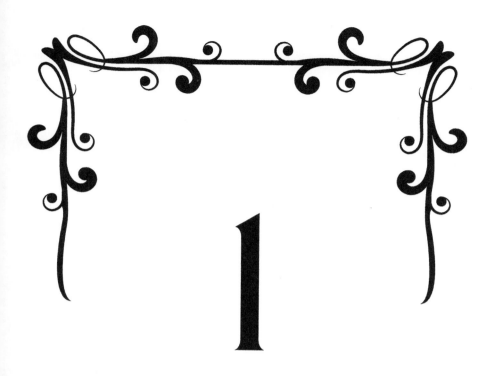

1

Mindful
Horticulture

Before I get into the nitty-gritty details to "set the stage" for sharing my trauma journey (see chapter four if you're anxious to get to that part), it is important that I explain the background and tenets behind what *mindful horticulture* is, so you can understand how I integrated it into my recovery, and now, my life. The concept of mindful horticulture is simple, but enveloping it wholly into your life takes commitment, discipline, and most of all, practice.

Towards the middle of 2019, I was referred to a psychotherapist who specializes in pain management. She is a huge believer in the power of mindfulness, and its positive impact on a patient's physical and mental well-being. I was extremely skeptical about mindfulness when it was first proposed to me. Prior to my brain injury, I had heard the expression "being mindful" during yoga classes, and from some of my physiotherapists (who wanted me to stop rushing through my exercises), but I never truly knew what it meant. I didn't understand the logic behind mindfulness; I thought they were asking me to turn my mind off, and ignore the screaming and frenetic thoughts in my brain. I also needed to get past the fact that the term always invokes the notion of meditation. My mind was, and is, too busy and distracted to get the full benefits of a meditation practice. I was too arrogant and too anxious to change my thought process around the concept of meditation. I needed to understand that meditation is one way of achieving mindfulness, but it's not the only way. It's amazing how a brain injury can make you re-evaluate how you understand and emotionally react to certain ideas. You are forced to shed arrogance, preconceived notions and expectations for yourself, and to be open-minded to different therapies that could help your recovery.

MINDFULNESS

The easiest way to define mindfulness is that it is the act of paying attention on purpose, without judgement, to the present moment. Wait a second, but that sounds easy? It is easy, for a few seconds at a time, but then our insanely busy minds take over and we get distracted. The goal is to reduce those distractions and to stay in the present moment, focusing on exactly what you're doing, down to the finest and most minute detail. The only way to achieve this state is with lots of practice. I still consider myself a beginner in the art of mindfulness. If you'd like to read about a true master, Thich Nhat Hanh is a famous Buddhist monk from Vietnam who fully embodies the meaning of mindfulness and its application to everyday tasks.[1] He has published over one hundred books teaching that mindfulness is a way of life, which anyone can achieve, regardless of their state of health, religion, race, sexuality, gender identity, or social status. It is a completely agnostic tool for self-care. While you may start out with only a few mindful moments every day, as you practice staying in the present, you can slowly progress to being mindful throughout the majority of the day, including times when you're doing menial tasks around the house, when you are having conversations with others, spending time with your family, etc. Aside from when you're reminiscing about the past or planning for the future, the rest of your day can be spent mindfully, without worry and with focus on intentional patience towards yourself and others.

A mindfulness practice forces you to acknowledge everything that is going on in your brain and environment. You aren't asked to change any of it, but you are asked to put the distractions aside while you're focusing on your task at hand. A mindful practice will help you develop compassion and kindness for yourself, your thoughts, and your environment, which will eventually allow you to get past all of the commotion that is so inherent in day-to-day life.

In full disclosure, before I discovered that it was possible to apply the action of "being mindful" to everyday activities, I tried to establish a meditation practice again. I read a lot of books because I felt like I had been doing it very, very wrong the first ten to twelve times that I'd tried it. One interesting thing that I learned was that "mindfulness meditation" is a non-concentrative technique; meaning that you aren't focusing on a single object, phrase, or sound. Being mindful in meditation entails opening your mind and widening your consciousness to the experience of meditating; the act of sitting quietly in reflective observation and subtly noticing the environment around you.[2] I gave meditation, on my own, as a silent practice the good ol' college try, but I got frustrated with the ease of which my brain veered into different directions, and how sitting still was (badly) hurting my back and neck (even with proper meditation pillows). The pain was a distraction all on its own. Not wanting to give up too quickly, I tried guided meditations, which would help refocus my meditative efforts. There are tons of free and paid apps for guided meditations. Some of the best ones include: Headspace, InsightTimer, and mySleepButton. My absolute favorite one though is 10% Happier; there is also a book of the same title written by Dan Harris, the face and founder of the app. His name might sound familiar because he is the ABC News anchor and correspondent who famously had a panic attack on national television.[3] After reading his book, I realized how much I identified with what he went through. We both have addictive personalities, overpowering negative voices in our heads that tell us we aren't achieving success unless we're full-out balls to the walls, and we prioritize our careers over every other aspect of our lives—including our health. I thought if meditation could work for him, then it should work for me!

I give myself an "A" for effort. I still continued with a guided meditation regime, but I only did it at night before bed to help calm and relax my mind. Seven times out of ten, I fell asleep before the end of the guided meditation. I consider that a win-win, even though it's not the point of meditating. I still needed to find a way that I could achieve mindfulness without having to be still. Mindfulness is supposed to be a powerful tool in pain management, just ask my therapist, but I couldn't achieve it when I was hurting too much to get past it. My next inspiration on my quest for a successful mindfulness technique was to consult Mr. Miyagi from *The Karate Kid*.

I really don't know what made me think about that movie, but I was reminiscing with my husband one day about how I used to have a crush on Ralph Macchio, despite our extreme age difference. I had just finished attempting to meditate, while sitting on my specifically designed meditation pillows, and every vertebrae in my back and neck were screaming at me. I had the beginnings of a tension headache. It was when Steve (my husband) said "wax on, wax off"—because that's one of the only things he remembered about the movie—when it clicked! Mr. Miyagi was trying to teach the karate kid how to obtain focus and mindfulness in the task at hand, in the present, by having him wax his vintage cars. Then I remembered when he also made him paint his fence with slow and deliberate strokes, and encouraged him to try to catch a fly with his chopsticks. All of these were acts that required mindfulness and focus in the present to achieve. How could I have been so blind? I didn't need to meditate to achieve mindfulness, it is just one way that works for some people. I could carry out my daily activities with more attention and focus with the intention of achieving a state of mindfulness. Now where to start?

I started with something that I knew better than I knew my own self. I started with the simplest, yet most irrefutable treasures of life. Coffee. I wrote the steps I wanted to take before I immersed myself in the process:

1. Smell the coffee before taking a sip;
2. Notice the different layers of the scent;
3. Take a sip and hold it in my mouth for a few seconds before swallowing it;
4. Taste and smell are intricately tied together. Could I resolve what I smelled with what I tasted?

These small acts of "noticing" and "being present," in this otherwise mundane activity, have allowed me to enjoy and savor my morning coffee moments more. It is taking a moment (even just a few seconds) for yourself, your brain, and being in the present . . . without judgement. You might even already be doing this when you drink coffee in the morning, not knowing that you're actually absorbed in the moment. You're present. You're mindful.

Mindfulness allows you to develop focus by establishing intentions and creating an outlet for you to direct your attention; this is why it is most easily achieved doing simple tasks, there are lots of methods and potential points of focus. Indoor horticulture, the cultivation and propagation of houseplants can be a mindful outlet. The only difference between task-oriented mindfulness and meditation is the fact that you're still moving your body. For people with chronic pain and brain trauma, movement is key for managing pain and maintaining concentration. In my opinion, achieving extended periods of mindfulness is the key to happiness; I am still in the process of being able to mindfully go throughout my day, however, one place where I can truly focus on the present and my self-care is when I am caring for my plants.

SELF-CARE IS NOT SELFISH

Before I go too far in describing the practice of mindful horticulture, I would like to take a moment to discuss self-care. Self-care is only one facet of the physical and mental health continuum. In North American society, this concept is quite new in relative terms. Self-care is the practice of deliberately taking care of your personal emotional, mental, and physical well-being.[4] Again, it seems like common sense, but it is one of the most overlooked elements within our daily lives. We've become so obsessed with our jobs, mortgages, paying bills, doing chores, and taking care of our kids, our significant others, and our extended families that we fail to address our need for setting aside time to care for ourselves.

As an example, you might enjoy running your kids to soccer practice, coaching the team, and then socializing with the parents, but are these self-care activities? Just because you enjoy something, doesn't necessarily mean that it's healthy for you physically and mentally. We, as a society, tend to consolidate activities that we enjoy and find fulfilling with self-care. They aren't always the same thing, and they aren't mutually exclusive of each other either. Eventually, if you maintain this pace and continue to disregard your needs, your gas tank will hit empty, and you'll need to find a way to re-engage with your well-being at the expense of some other task or activity. Classic burnout. Having a regular self-care regime allows you to refuel yourself, so you can perform better as a human being, complete every-day tasks, and take care of others. Self-care needs to be something that is specifically planned in your schedule, it can't be something that "just happens," and it needs to be responsive to your current mental and physical health needs. For some people, running and going to the gym is their self-care regime. For others, it is reading a book. Sometimes you can have multiple components to your self-care regime. What works to re-energize and re-invigorate me, might not work for others.

Self-care is not a substitute for medical or psycho-therapeutic treatment; it is complementary to the treat-ment plan that you map out with your health care pro-viders. Both self-care and mindfulness were prescribed by my therapist as separate and unique entities. I have since learned that they can be combined, as working to attain a state of mindfulness is a form of self-care. Mindfulness can improve your interactions with your health care providers by making you more receptive and aware of your symptoms. Mindfulness is a way of life, not just something you try in times of crisis; aim for it to be incorporated into your everyday, not just a transient part of treatment. It is a life-long commitment, but is worth the practice, time, and effort.

I am a work in progress in terms of mapping time for myself. My brain has issues wrapping itself around the idea that "me time" is not a waste of time. In my past life, I was obsessed with efficiency, perfection, and performance; those are hard habits to break. I rationalize my time with my plants as being both good for me and good for them; it helps take the edge off the anxiety I feel when I worry that I'm taking too much "me time." Eventually I hope to get to the point where just taking care of myself is reason enough to justify the time that I spend on self-care. Like I said, I'm a work in progress.

MINDFUL HORTICULTURE AS A PRACTICE

Horticulture therapy is a recognized mental health treatment strategy. It is defined as using plants and gardening activities as tools in professionally conducted programs of therapy and rehabilitation.[5] When most people think of horticulture they think of gardening and agriculture. Unfortunately, our cold Canadian climate restricts these outdoor activities to less than half the year. If we open our minds to more, we can see the year-round benefits of indoor horticulture to extend our therapy. It doesn't mean that we have to build giant greenhouses to facilitate horticulture therapy, we can get our hands dirty and gain the benefits of a gardening practice indoors with a single potted plant. In Canada, there are very few registered horticulture therapists simply because it is an emerging field of mental and physical health therapy. At the moment there are a limited number of training courses that are acknowledged by the Canadian Horticulture Therapy Association. With the resurgence in popularity of house plants and gardening with millennials, this is sure to change.

Through guided and supervised tasks using living material that requires human intervention for optimal survival, a horticulture therapist can assess, evaluate, and positively contribute to a patient's physical well-being, cognition and perception, emotional well-being, and social skills. The achievement of mindfulness through horticulture is just one benefit of the horticulture therapy technique. Mindful horticulture is a self-care tool that can be used by anyone, you don't need to be trained in therapeutic horticulture, and you don't need to have a traumatic brain injury or a mental health diagnosis to benefit from living and being present with plants. I reiterate that mindful horticulture as a self-care practice is not a replacement or substitute for professional counseling or psychotherapy. It is complementary.

Mindful horticulture can be applied to both indoor and outdoor gardens. This practice involves slowing down your thoughts, tending to your plants in an organized and intentional way, noticing any changes in their health (both positive and negative), and recognizing when they require augmentation to their soil, light, water, or nutrient levels. It is about moving intentionally through the care of your plants while noticing how it is making you feel. If a negative emotion or sensation arises, acknowledge its presence, allow yourself to move past the emotion or sensation and continue working through the activity. This practice should be gentle, both physically and mentally. Be aware of your limitations. If you need to work while sitting down, move all of your plants and tools to a bench or table before starting your focused practice, rather than finding everything haphazardly and inducing pain while continually repositioning your body. The small act of noticing new growth, the hardening off of a new leaf, or seeing new roots sprout from the bottom of a pot can be very therapeutic, incredibly inspiring, and can positively contribute to a sense of purpose.

When I am working with my plants, I am trying to obtain comfort in a state of silence. As an introvert, my energy levels are refreshed in quiet spaces. I don't listen to music or watch videos when I'm working with my plants. I'm not capable of obtaining the level of easy and natural focus required to have a state of mindfulness with those types of auditory distractions. Everyone is different though, some people find music helps to center and focus their intentions.

MINDFUL HORTICULTURE JOURNALING

My journaling practice started following my brain injury. I would have "Good Brain Days" and "Bad Brain Days," and I needed to record the differences between them, so I could recognize and appreciate the days that were better than others. Regardless of whether you have experienced trauma, injury, or issues with mental health, everyone has good brain days and bad brain days. When my sister was pregnant with my nephew, she'd have days when she was "foggy." Her memory would be bad, she put dishes in the freezer and couldn't string words into a sentence. These are exactly the types of days when journaling would be a useful tool to figure out what was different in how you approached the day, if you ate a meal at a different time, if you woke up with a headache, etc. For myself, I needed to understand how I was caring for myself differently day-to-day in order to isolate behaviors that would allow me to have more good brain days going forward in my recovery. Actively keeping a journal helped me understand I was responsible and had control over most things that influenced whether I had a good brain day or not. First I noticed, the good days always started out with some alone time with my plants. As I became more aware of the benefits of mindfulness, I would incorporate that into my plant-care practice. Second, I realized that being purposefully active first thing in the morning would set me up both physically and mentally to have a good day. I always felt better on the days when I would start out being centered, active, and present. That discovery completely changed my personal outlook for my post-injury recovery. Since then, my journaling has evolved to become a record of both my mindfulness practice and my urban jungle journey.

I have found journaling to be beneficial for three reasons: first, it allows you to plan your self-care practice; second, it allows you to retroactively think about what you experienced during your practice and understand how you dealt with each emotion or feeling (positive or negative) at the time, so you can learn from that reflection; finally, journaling allows you to look back and have a written record of how far you've come. Has achieving mindfulness become easier? Are you able to get past negative emotions in order to remain present in the activity? If not, how can you tweak your practice to include more compassion for yourself?

Journaling does not have to be exhaustive, particularly if you don't enjoy writing. The first journal that I kept was completely for practical purposes; it was a record of all the plants in my collection, when they came into my care, and some notes on their care requirements. It took me a long time to find a format I liked for my journaling that was simple and elegant, while being functional. I also didn't want to use an excel spreadsheet for this activity because it is so impersonal; my plants are like my friends, they aren't numbers in a spreadsheet. The act of handwriting everything out about each individual plant allows me to feel like I'm taking ownership of their survival, with the understanding that some loss is inevitable as it is a learning process. This collection record should be personal and tailored to your needs. There are commercial products out there for this activity, but it isn't necessary to spend money on a fancy journal to reap the benefits of documenting your jungle. I am a plant collector; I love the rare and exotic, so it only makes sense that I would want to have a record of each individual plant; my plants are investments, they are my base plant stock for future propagations. I want to share my passion with the rest of the Canadian plant community. Documenting their care instructions and noting any quirks in their cultivation makes this information easier to pass on.

The second and third journaling activities that I do are specifically focused on my mindful horticulture practice. These journaling activities are one hundred percent complementary to each other, and I have included some example journal pages in Appendix 1 and 2. The weekly planner and daily journal were created to help you prioritize your self-care within your daily routine. Life gets busy. The practice of planning your self-care *before* your practice will allow you to slow down and check in with yourself. The practice of journaling about your experience *afterwards* will permit you to pay attention and stay purposefully in the present with kindness and curiosity while maintaining your garden. Moving forward, you can journal with the intent to recognize what you observed and the emotions you experienced.

The prompts that are provided within the daily journal are a starting place for your mindful horticulture practice. You are invited to connect with your body, heart, mind, environment, and the relationship that you have with your plants. Feel free to fill out each section, or don't. Pick the sections that resonate the most with you. If you feel that there are other questions or prompts that you would like to include, ensure they will serve to deepen your self-awareness, inspire insight, and empower your choices.

This act of planning and post-practice journaling shouldn't take longer than ten minutes every day. Do it just for you and discover how a mindful horticulture practice can be beneficial to your recovery and overall mental health. These are just tips and tricks to help you on your way. Find what works for you. Mindful horticulture is not the only mindful self-care practice that I employ; at night I meditate before going to sleep, to settle my brain; I also love the sun (of course fully sunscreened because I'm a super pale northerner), some of my most transcendent mindfulness experiences are when I close my eyes and put my face up to the sun for a few moments, enjoying the heat and brightness, breathing in the warmed air, and noticing the change in temperature. This is very surreal for me. Try it sometime.

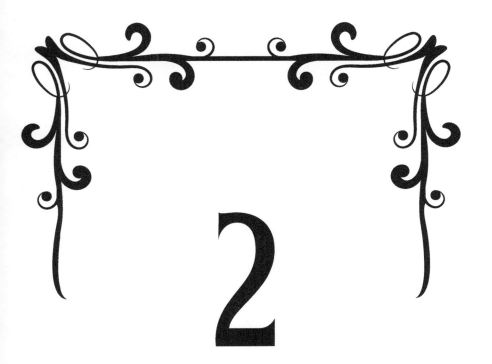

2

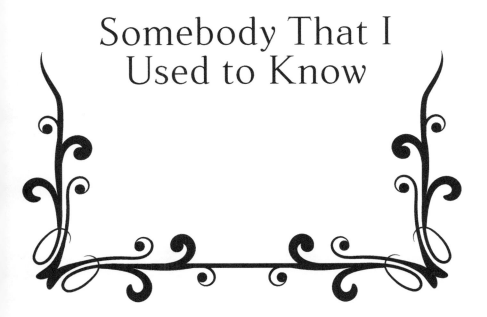

Somebody That I Used to Know

I didn't know it at the time, but my journey to find mindful horticulture started well before my traumatic brain injury. Without my previous history, the challenges and the successes, my recovery story would have been different. I would like to share my entire story with you, in the hopes that you'll benefit from some of the discoveries I made, or even see yourself in some of my past experiences. Everyone recovers from trauma differently, but it's amazing to note how much influence the past has on how we deal with grief, pain, and loss. I hope that sharing my journey will invite others to learn from my experiences and open lines of communication, empathy, and insight into the little known worlds of trauma, brain injury, and mental health.

This chapter is the most difficult part of my story to tell; not because it is overly emotional, but because I have lost quite a bit of it to the abyss of my brain injury; a lot of my memories are fuzzy. When I was young, I prided myself on having an exceptional memory. Before the era of digital cameras in our phones, I used to get irritated when people would make me stop what I was doing to capture a moment on film. Taking pictures wasn't something that I valued. I always thought I'd just remember the experience and that would be a thousand times better than looking at a 2D photo. That's one of my greatest regrets. I have so many memories that are lost and unrecoverable. It is important to explain my life before my concussion, so you'll understand exactly why I went through a significant period of mourning, self-hatred, and profound depression post-injury.

I grew up like most kids in the 1980s. I had a nuclear family—two parents and two siblings (both younger). My parents didn't divorce until I was in my late teens, after I'd already left home. Divorce wasn't as common or accepted back then. I didn't realize how different my family experience was until after my parents separated and I had left home. Under the veil of matrimony (pun intended), problems are easily hidden from the outside world rendering a picture perfect family to the unwitting observer. In all honesty, I thought everyone's parents spoke to each other the way my parents did. I didn't know that passive-aggressive condescension and yelling weren't normal behaviors. I understood that every kid looked forward to one of their parents being away, so they could relax and let their guard down with the remaining parent. Didn't everyone have to snap to attention, be better behaved and pseudo-scared when dad got home? Didn't every mom ask their kids to keep secrets from their dad about the activities they did without him, or the money spent in his absence? Growing up, I accepted that this was normal in our family; and I seriously thought everyone else's family dynamic was the same.

I am originally from a small town in southern Alberta, and was then transplanted outside of Winnipeg, Manitoba just prior to my grade eleven year. Small towns are hard to escape if you don't have the motivation to be bigger than your origin. It was my observation at the time that the further away your small town of origin was from a decent-sized city, the less likely you were to leave. Staying was not an option for me. The military was something different, an opportunity that none of my peers were interested in, and it would be an adventure—it was my ticket out. While I'm grateful that I grew up in a small town and had all the rural experiences, I was never going to stay after high school. I had huge expectations for myself. Joining the Canadian Armed Forces (CAF) at seventeen, was a natural fit for my internal-turned-external escapist. My desire to break free had a lot to do with my dad.

Dad and I had a very odd, stressful, and complicated relationship; it was my perception when I was younger that my dad and I were in constant competition, in every way. Whether it was in sports or if my science project was inferior to one that he had done in his youth, he was always better. It was a relationship of trying to *one-up* each other under the guise he was trying to give me a multitude of experiences and encouraging me to be the best. Instead, it felt like I was never good enough; I always had to find ways to better myself to (misguidedly) impress him. If I transcended him at something, he was angry, if I didn't, he was disappointed, and expressed both feelings readily. Dad is a civil engineer. Where we lived, that type of education and achievement was rare. He was one-of-one in his job and he was incredibly ostentatious. Dad was very proud of his status in town, and imposed himself on town council as a councilman, and volunteered at the fire department to inflate his standing. Of course, I didn't realize any of this was a personality flaw, I worshiped him and needed to have his approval at all costs. He was a narcissist and he did his very best to turn me into a compliant clone.

I knew that I wanted to attend the Royal Military College of Canada (RMC) for engineering from the time I was seven years old. On a formative trip near Kingston, ON to visit my paternal grandparents, we went on an outing to the Fort Henry tourist attraction, which overlooks the RMC peninsula. As I stood on the ringed booster ledge of the sightseeing scope looking out over the college's limestone buildings, I overheard my dad casually say that he had applied to attend RMC, but hadn't gotten in because he didn't have the right academic or extracurricular background. He went on to say that RMC was where all the elite, the best-of-the-best men went to school and that it was very difficult to get in. At that exact moment, I knew that I had to attend. His statement about his failure to get into RMC was a sign of weakness that I could exploit. Thankfully, the military had already started the integration of women into the RMC population in 1984, so I wasn't limited by my gender.

I was expected to go to a university that he coveted, to become an engineer because not being an engineer was not an option. It was an unspoken expectation, passive-aggressively hinted at throughout my childhood. One of the Topping children would be an engineer; it was non-negotiable and that child would be me. Other professions were inferior.

Years of psychotherapy and the experience of writing this all out, has made me realize our relationship was incredibly unhealthy. I have only recently extricated myself from my sense of obligation to him. Dad and I are now estranged, and I don't have any regrets. Sometimes toxic relationships aren't worth maintaining when they are at the expense of your personal health and happiness. As an adult, it took a long time to realize that I get to decide who is in my life and who isn't.

Joining the military and going to RMC fit my personality at the time. Very early on I had started to purposefully curate my academic and extracurricular activities, so I would be a perfect candidate for my chosen career path. I was an air cadet, participated in every sport possible in my school, held leadership positions, and achieved scholastically in all the requisite courses. I barely had time to breathe as a kid, but I had a clear goal. I trained myself to do things that didn't come naturally to me; looking people in the eye when I spoke to them, engaging in conversations with new adults, and speaking confidently. I molded myself to be the perfect candidate for military college. I was so single-minded in my efforts that I only applied to one other university, in the event I didn't get into RMC. It was my "safety university," and it was the most undesirable option I could imagine: the University of Manitoba, in engineering (of course), and living at home. I would have been emotionally destroyed if I didn't get into RMC and had my entire future riding on receiving that specific acceptance letter.

RMC is one of the last universities in Canada to send out acceptance letters; it was agonizing watching all of my peers receive their letters; and listening to them talk about whether they would go away to school or stay close to home. The majority of them opted to stay near home and to live with their parents. I didn't get it, and was secretly disgusted with the thought of sitting at home for four more years. As my dad always said, it wasn't fiscally responsible for me to consider leaving home unless I was on a full-ride scholarship. I needed to prove to him I could do it. The wait gave me such an overwhelming sense of trepidation and anxiety that I felt like I was drowning. This feeling wasn't good anticipation; it was almost like watching your potential future on a slow motion reel and the scenes begin to spontaneously combust until there is almost nothing left.

* * *

My acceptance letter to RMC to study engineering came in early April. The flood of relief I felt is indescribable. The weight of worry lifted, and I felt like I could accomplish anything.

The military was a gateway for me to achieve all the expectations I had for myself. I loved the Basic Officer Training Course (BOTC), it is a twelve-week long indoctrination into military life, leadership training, and learning how to push yourself past your perceived limits. Lucky for me, my experience as an air cadet was integral in ensuring that minor military tasks—like polishing boots, relearning how to march (drill), and ironing uniforms—didn't drag me down as I was playing the rest of the indoctrination game. By the time I got to

BOTC, I was so relieved that everything had worked out and that I had gained my independence.

Then came the dreaded six-week RMC Recruit Term; I heard horror stories from fellow trainees and it sounded like an absolute nightmare. My anxiety would peak and I'd break into a cold sweat whenever I overheard folks talking about it. It was a barely controlled and monitored form of hazing with a bit of psychological warfare thrown in for good measure; thanks to the combination of the worst aspects of basic training (waking up well before the sun, being yelled at, and having a schedule so jam-packed you barely had time to pee), attending university courses, and the people in charge of recruit term were just *kids* only a few years older than the students. At the time, the goal of recruit term, much like BOTC, is to break down all of your personal barriers (both physical and mental) and to rebuild you into a confident, model cadet. I didn't make it out of recruit term unscathed; it was my first introduction to real, heartbreaking failure, and RMC was a complete and total culture shock.

There are four pillars of excellence at RMC, which all cadets have to succeed in to graduate; in no particular order they are: leadership, academics, athletics, and bilingualism.

Leadership is hard to evaluate until you're not the scum-sucking, bottom-feeder at the lowest end of the hierarchy. I thought I'd have at least academics and athletics easily licked—I couldn't have been more wrong. Nearing the end of recruit term, I had failed all of my midterms in first semester, except for English and psychology—I was seriously contemplating my future as the next generation engineer in my family; I couldn't understand why things didn't come as easily to me as they had in high school. It took me a few weeks to realize that I was surrounded by people just like me—they had gotten into RMC on the same merits that I did. Everything at RMC is super-charged because our schedules are maxed out; we have insane deadlines; huge personal and institutional expectations laid upon us; we are ALL THE SAME, we are all silently competing amongst each other and sorting out our new social hierarchy.

I almost quit until I found *my people*—a couple of older gentlemen, at least they seemed old at the time, although they were probably in their late twenties, early thirties (maybe) who had past military experience. I would have never made it out of my first year without them. They recognized that I was out of my depth after midterms and they took me under their wing. These guys made me sit in the front row with them and re-focused my attention onto academics. They saved me from drowning at the expense of my immaturity and arrogance. I pulled up my socks and made it past those early academic failures—I graduated from RMC having never had to write a supplemental exam in any of my academic courses, a minor miracle.

The bilingualism requirement was a whole different ball game. I, unfortunately, was in French class all four years of RMC. French language courses were not an option in my small school in Alberta, and since I was years behind my peers by the time I moved to

Manitoba, I opted out as it would have dropped my GPA too much to try it. French training is mandatory at RMC and for those who aren't bilingual, there are five hours of class a week, plus homework. A little pity from the second language testing agent and some pre-exam alcohol were necessary for me to be considered "functionally" bilingual before graduation.

When it came to athletics, it took me until second year to figure out where I belonged. In high school, I had always played sports because I knew that they would be part of the *complete* application package when I applied for RMC. With a natural aptitude for team sports, I was usually one of the better players on the field or court, but I completely lacked passion. I was coordinated, flexible, and in decent shape, but I was only mediocre at the mandatory RMC physical fitness tests. In my first year, I attempted volleyball and basketball. I was cut from the volleyball team, then I broke my ankle during a basketball game, which ended athletics completely for that year. In second year, I ran into the captain of the varsity women's rugby team at the Snake Pit, the cadet bar, during the first week back at school; she was actively recruiting people to come try out for the team. I had never heard of rugby before; she guaranteed that I would love the sport. Trying out for the rugby team was the absolute best decision I ever made. I instantly fell in love with the sport. Our team was TERRIBLE compared to the other university teams, but it didn't matter, we were a team. I got out a lot of pent up frustration and aggression on the rugby pitch. It was an outlet for me, and I met some of the most amazing people. To this day, I'm still in contact with my very first rugby coach.

For the rest of my time at RMC, during rugby season, I ate, slept, and breathed rugby. It was my obsession. It wouldn't be uncommon for the professor to find my teammates and I with our heads together over a workbook coming up with set plays, line-ups, and lineouts during a lecture. We were a team that practiced and played rugby together, but like all rugby clubs, we also partied together. During the fall season, you couldn't talk to me unless it was related to rugby because I was intensely focused on the upcoming practice, game, or beer-up. The women on the rugby team were the single reason I loved my time at RMC so much—unfortunately, it was also the start of all my current health problems.

I played rugby at RMC from 1999 to 2002; it was a completely different time with respect to how any on-pitch injury is treated now. There were two relevant and unwritten tenets of RMC life that I've failed to mention to this point: 1) pain is just weakness leaving the body, suck it up; and 2) going to the cadet medical infirmary unless you're dying of the plague, have a broken limb, or a dental emergency, is akin to committing social suicide. No one wanted to be labeled a medical commando. Interestingly enough, my dad had much the same philosophy when I was growing up, so it was easy enough for me to "drink the (proverbial) Kool-aid."

Being pulled off the pitch in the middle of a rugby match for an injury was also not an option. If someone was the best player for that position, regardless of injury, we weren't encouraged to take a knee. I've witnessed scrum halves play with broken fingers, an outside center playing with a badly sprained ankle, and forwards playing with dislocated shoulders. You have to be a particular type of crazy to buy into rugby culture. I was exactly that type of crazy.

In the coaches' defence, back then not much was known about the effects of concussions and sports-related head injuries. I remember four distinct occasions where my brain was rattled around so badly that I had difficulty functioning day-to-day afterwards. The effects usually only lasted three to five days so I wasn't too concerned about it. On three of the four occasions, I never told a living soul that I felt unwell, that I couldn't play or practice, or that I was suffering in any way. Part of it was stubbornness, but a lot of it was social stigma, and just me not wanting to be *that* person that was injured again. Breaking my ankle in my first year was an eye-opener to the criticism and disgrace that an injured person faced while at the college. I was in a cast, on crutches in the middle of winter, but I still felt the disdain from my peers. I have definitely teased a few people for having to take a knee, so I know that I was part of the problem—particularly when I became a senior member of the team in fourth year. I was put in my place later that year though during the second to last game of our season, I was kicked in the face so hard while trying to remove myself from the bottom of a collapsed ruck that my nose broke. Blood spewed everywhere and I saw those bright flashes of light that everyone talks about following a head injury. I literally felt my brain smash into the back of my skull and then go careening into the front of it. I blacked out for a short-enough period of time that no one noticed anything except the splatters of blood.

The physiotherapist checked my face; my nose was obviously broken because it was at a very unattractive angle, but my level of consciousness and ability to cognitively function were not assessed at all. The therapists and coaches knew that I would put up a fight to finish the game. I had a particular reputation for never wanting to come off the pitch and for being fairly argumentative about it if it were suggested—the physiotherapists *knew* better. So, aside from cutting a tampon in two and putting one piece up each side of my nose to staunch the bleeding, they carried out no concussion diagnoses and I continued playing.

After the game (which we lost terribly), I went to the emergency room only to have my nose reset—and again, no concussion protocol was carried out because I didn't tell anyone that there was a problem. In the meantime, I had a raging headache, a nauseous feeling in the pit of my stomach, and was completely unable to focus on anything that anyone was saying to me. I was more worried about getting out of the ER in time to attend the after-game beer call than I was about receiving proper treatment. The next two weeks were an absolute nightmare; I had difficulty concentrating, bouts of falling asleep inappropriately in class (which was out of character for me), dizziness, and a lack of appetite—all symptoms of a concussion. I attributed it to the amount of over-the-counter pain relievers I was using for my throbbing nose. I still attended every rugby practice (although I couldn't play), every class, and participated in military activities—life went on. I struggled for the rest of the fall semester and didn't take any time to recover until the Christmas break. Luckily, I returned to RMC in January feeling much better, however, there were persistent changes in my personality. I also had a falling out with one of my closest college friends. It took so much effort to maintain my mostly stable status quo that I couldn't maintain our friendship after I indirectly witnessed her having a mean girl moment to people who didn't deserve her wrath and indifference. Losing her friendship resulted in a complete change in my social circle during my last months at the college. It was a gruelling time.

In the spring of 2002, while we were gearing up to practice for the graduation parade, it was announced that the RMC Women's Varsity Rugby Team was disbanded; the team was seen as taking too much of the scarcely available female population (it took thirty women to field a rugby team and there were only about 225 of us total, at the college), and there were too many injuries that were affecting military occupation training (our future military careers were at stake). The really crushing part was that they were going to keep and maintain a men's rugby team. I have never been so mad in my entire life; I saw red. The injustice of it all was overwhelming! I had already played out my years of rugby, but it wouldn't be an option for the younger members of the team or even future recruits. Even my younger sister, Carrie, had played rugby when she started at the college two years after I did. Our team's legacy, however unsuccessful, was over. I couldn't imagine life at the college without the rugby team. While I understood the logistics of the administration's decision, it still felt like an unfair, sexist, kick to the teeth. It wasn't until I returned to RMC four years later to do my masters, that I not-so-delicately insisted that the concept of reinstating the team be revisited with the RMC athletic and administrative bodies.

As cliché as it sounds, I wouldn't be the person I am today if I hadn't attended RMC, if I hadn't taken the leap to leave my prairie small town behind, and if I hadn't played on that rugby team. My most formative years that shaped who I am as an adult, took place on that peninsula. I grew up at RMC and will be eternally grateful for the experience.

* * *

There is a general understanding within the military community that officers who graduated from RMC have an attitude—a sense of entitlement—when they enter the regular military workforce. We are all ring-knockers who seize every opportunity to remind subordinates that we went to RMC, and get to hob-nob with senior officers who are also alumni. I was warned very early in my summer training about this distasteful reputation that would invariably be bestowed on me. A sergeant I encountered in the summer of 2000 took me aside and told me not to be an asshole, that my subordinates were my best asset, and that they could and would make or break my career. To this day, that is the best advice I've ever gotten. I like to think I started out my military career on the right foot because that sergeant had enough respect for me to explain the what's what and who's who.

After RMC and my last phase of aerospace engineering training (my assigned military occupation), I had a very unconventional career; most young officers go to field units to get their first taste of military life, not me! I went to a military research facility in Toronto and worked on state-of-the-art aerospace life support equipment projects. This posting set the stage for the rest of my twenty-two year career. To quell my thirst for knowledge, I started my master's in environmental engineering, part-time, taking courses at the University of Toronto. The warrant officer and civilian, who worked directly for me in the shop, expertly guided me and molded me to be their ideal supervisor. I used to joke they were literally my right and left hands, I couldn't get anything done without them. The major in charge of the entire shop let me run with ideas and gave me the freedom to make mistakes in order to learn from them. I couldn't have asked for a better team to work with, and for, during my first posting experience.

As a young twenty-one-year-old officer, Toronto was an ideal posting. I loved having a packed work, academic, and social calendar, and being in control of more of my life. I continued to play rugby recreationally while I was in Toronto. While I've grown to dislike the big city, I enjoyed it before the daily gridlock, crush of people, and never-ending noise jaded me; it was something I had to do while I was young. Toronto was both overwhelming and completely liberating.

The busier I was, the more the little voice in my head was telling me I wasn't working hard enough or that I was disappointing people. I didn't recognize it, but I was spiralling. I became obsessed with being the best at my job, the best in school, the best in my recreational activities, and maintaining a specific level of perfection. These obsessive-compulsive traits were regulated while I was at RMC, under someone's thumb, but as soon as I was *in control* they manifested into an unhealthy pattern. It all started with a rugby injury and deteriorated from there.

As I've demonstrated, I've always been incredibly competitive. I joined a rugby team outside of the Greater Toronto Area because I had heard amazing things about the coach, the playing facilities, and the athlete development program. It seemed worth the hour drive to participate, but little did I know, I was joining a team that looked super cohesive (from the outside), but once you were in, it was like high school all over again! I jumped in with both feet, determined to overcome the social drama that the central clique created and get past the stigma of being a *transient* (an unfortunate side effect of military life). I just wanted to play rugby—my goal was to obtain a highly coveted position on the first side. So, I played and practiced hard—extremely hard. I didn't report the first, second, or even tenth time that my shoulder would subluxate or dislocate. I was in extreme pain, but the continued dislocations meant that my shoulder joint became looser and looser, rendering it easier and easier to put it back in place myself . . . until I couldn't. In 2004, my shoulder eventually gave out and I had to go see a doctor; my problem was way worse than requiring just a few sessions of physiotherapy—I needed surgery. This pattern of sucking it up until things were so bad that I needed serious medical intervention was a consequence of my own feelings of inadequacy, ingrained environmental triggers, and an unhealthy competitive streak. Injuries and delayed medical treatment, like what happened to my shoulder, didn't happen just once, but repeatedly throughout my career. I have had four, soon to be five, surgeries to fix chronic joint and bone conditions that I let fester to the point of disability.

In the wake of shoulder surgery, I was overcome with a sense of uselessness, despair, and loneliness. I don't really know how it started, but I began consuming alcohol as a way of controlling my inner demons, and to pass the time. Prior to this injury, I had a healthy appetite for booze, but would only drink in excess socially and never when I was alone. The military and rugby both have an overlying drinking culture, so I was sucked into the habit quite organically, as awful as that sounds. Despite being on medical leave, I went to work almost every day just so I wouldn't be home by myself. I would go to work and physiotherapy by day, everything seemed normal, but I would go home to a six-pack of Keith's every night and a couple of vodka chasers to help me sleep. From the outside looking in, I appeared to be so intent on having a successful recovery that I was approved to do the military physical fitness test just six weeks after surgery so I could go play softball in a military competition.

Despite the supportive nature of my chain-of-command, I still felt the social stigma associated with going to the medical community for help. I had an ingrained distrust for anyone in scrubs or with MD behind their name. Mental health was not something that was easily spoken about within the military community in the early 2000s. It wasn't until the Afghanistan War and the post-deployment aftermath of soldiers returning with operational stress injuries and post-traumatic stress disorder that the taboo slowly started to ease at a snail's pace. In early 2006, I self-identified as having a drinking problem and recognized that I was self-medicating in an attempt to alleviate my on-going crisis. I didn't tell anyone that I had a drinking problem, I quit cold turkey under the guise of wanting to lose weight—alcohol had empty calories. To my credit I haven't had a drink in over fourteen years, but at that point in time, I still didn't seek professional help. I thought self-identifying meant that I was stronger and more self-aware of my issues than other people were. Not true at all. My desire for control manifested in controlling my environment. I can literally follow my progression through unhealthy obsessive control mechanisms in the face of having an undiagnosed mental health problem. I am one hundred percent convinced that the concussions I experienced in my very early twenties contributed to my unstable mental health. Despite everything, I was promoted to captain that year and lost my *newbie* lustre.

I applied to go back to RMC to do my master's program full-time for a post-graduate training position. In preparation to go back, I started a weight-loss and exercise regime. I wanted to go back in great shape so I could fight to restart the women's rugby program, and so I would be a positive example for the cadets I would eventually teach. As per my norm, I took the situation to an unreasonable extreme. I started training for a marathon, despite not having run over three kilometers since leaving college. While I was training, I had this distorted notion that I was too heavy, and I was causing my body terrible damage by being so big. As a consequence, I started calorie counting. I lost more than fifty pounds in three months. I looked like a skeleton, but loved buying clothes that were a size four. I reveled in the fact that people were noticing my weight loss and how fit I was becoming. Their encouragement spurred me to work harder at the gym. I developed severe body dysmorphia, which still festers today.

Thankfully, a posting message arrived, and my life was taken over by moving to Kingston and starting school full-time, and I became distracted integrating into the post-graduate community. I still ran four marathons that year, but was less focused on my diet and I gradually reached a healthier, steady weight. I only had a year to finish my master's before I was due to be flung straight into carrying a full teaching load as a military lecturer. I didn't realize at the time, but this was taking me farther away from my intended military occupation.

In the summer of 2007, I completed my master's and began my lecturer position. I worked to be the best professor possible; since I struggled through my time as a cadet at RMC, I had a unique opportunity to connect with the cadets that not many professors did. I believe that if my health hadn't deteriorated how it did, I would have considered teaching as a viable post-military career choice. At the same time, I also took on coaching the newly revived RMC women's rugby club.

Word got around that I was a decent professor after the first year, so my teaching load increased. I still felt I wasn't engaged enough and enrolled myself in the doctorate program for chemical engineering. I didn't understand what being too busy meant. I was always juggling at least one too many things at a time. To be honest, I don't know why I applied for my doctorate; I hated lab work and I was a renowned procrastinator when it came to publishing results. However, I liked the idea of influencing scientific advancement, and I had HUGE ideas, but I wanted other people to do the grunt work. I had to put in my time as a student and postdoctoral fellow before I could reach that level of autonomy. Another factor that was always in the back of my mind was that I still really enjoyed one-upping my dad, who didn't have a postgraduate degree. I was the first in my family to get a master's with my sister following my footsteps several years later. Perhaps it would have been a defining moment once I completed my doctorate that would put me that extra step ahead of my father?

The end of the 2008 academic year was interesting. My students nominated me for the RMC Class of 1965 Teaching Excellence Award. This award is one of the most well-known, prestigious, and coveted prizes among the RMC Academic Wing. The award is endowed by the RMC Foundation and was initiated by the RMC Class of 1965 as a way to give back to the college through the recognition of excellence in teaching. Being nominated for this accolade was completely out of the blue, totally unexpected. I was only in my second year of teaching. This student-elected award is the pinnacle of anyone's teaching career if they are a professor who is there for their students, not just the research. When I was a cadet, I was lucky enough to have two professors who had won this award; they were heads and tails above the rest of the faculty.

To be considered in the same league as those professors was unbelievably flattering. It was even more astonishing when I won the award—never in a million years did I think I would win. It was like taking a long sweet drink of validation as a reward for the endless hours I put into delivering those courses.

A few of the other professors in the department joked that I had peaked too soon, and my teaching career was all downhill from there. Challenge accepted, I doubled down. I took on even more courses the next year, with larger class sizes, I continued to coach the rugby team, pushed to earn my doctorate, and I started training for an extreme physical challenge called the Petawawa Ironman (a four-stage military marathon). I think once I'd felt content that I was besting my dad, I needed to prove something to the rest of the world, too—I was setting myself up for a complete burn-out.

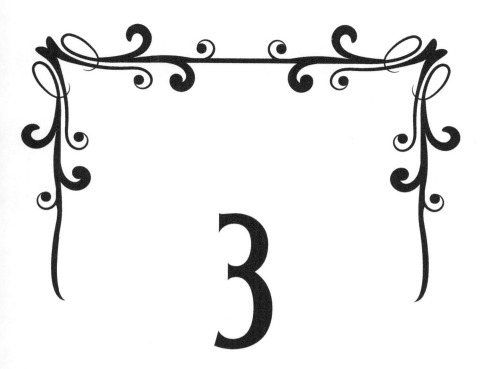

3

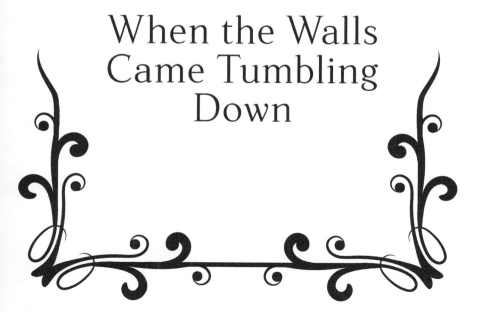

When the Walls Came Tumbling Down

My burnouts are monumental. They are slow burns that start with a busy schedule, turning into infernos when you add in the pressure associated with integrating into multiple social dynamics (academia, teaching, and rugby). Deep-seated feelings of personal inadequacy and hopelessness are further fuel for the fire. The cumulative stress that ultimately leads to one of my burnouts takes years to manifest until it volcanically erupts in my (and everyone else's) face. Go big or go home. That's how I am in life and in burnout. If you ask me what my life looked like before my concussion in 2016, I would tell you it was a revolving door of manic highs where I was succeeding and efficiently achieving, until I ultimately would peak-out and spiral into a deep depression. The manic high wouldn't come on like flipping a switch, rather it would ramp up slowly over time, sustaining itself with my inability to achieve less than perfection and need to please other people. Then BAM! I'd be down for the count, drowning in despair—numb. Everyday was the worst day of my life when I was on the other side of the revolving door.

Over the course of my post-graduate career, my doctorate advisor, who had also been my master's advisor, had become a father figure to me. He was the first supervisor I ever had who noticed that I wasn't doing well, mentally. He asked me on numerous occasions if a doctorate was something that I actually wanted, or if it was just another feather in my cap. I appreciated his concern, but misconstrued his meaning and thought he was insinuating that I couldn't do it, or I wasn't smart enough. Finally, he suggested that I apply for the military full-time doctorate position that had become available for the 2010 academic year, so I could focus more attention on my studies. In theory, it was a brilliant idea.

I applied for the position, and gratefully was accepted. Again, the plan was that once I'd finished my doctorate, I would be slated back into a faculty position to continue as a professor. I'm unsure what happened between June and September 2010, but I somehow got wrangled into teaching a course over the summer, which led to another course in the fall semester and yet another one in the winter. I didn't know how to say NO. I also didn't want to give up the courses I was teaching to someone else who wouldn't care as much about the cadets. I had developed something of a hero complex where I thought I was the only one who could do it and it needed to be done. In the process, my efforts kept being validated, as I was promoted to major in 2011. I continued to move further away from my intended career path based on my military occupation, and I was completely fine with that. I was riding the manic high again.

My expectations monumentally imploded in 2013 when I was informed that I was being posted away from RMC. This caught me off guard because I had received a posting message a few months earlier outlining that I was staying at RMC in a faculty position. It is the military though—they gave, and they take away.

My career manager informed me I had been away from my trade for too long and that there was a priority position that needed to be filled. Any delusions of self-importance that I had about filling a niche role in the CAF were shattered when I was told the real reason why I was the person being moved instead of other RMC personnel in similar positions of the same rank; I was the most "unencumbered" as I didn't have a family, I wasn't married, and I couldn't come up with a compassionate reason to stay in Kingston. I had never felt more betrayed by the military than I did at that exact moment. I felt like a convenient target, being that nobody needed me. I understood that, by joining the military, I signed on the dotted line and I was their tool to move around where the "powers that be" see fit. It wasn't until that exact moment though, that I realized that I was just a number, a *bum in a seat*. None of my accomplishments to that point meant anything. The disillusionment hit hard, and I had a complete meltdown. My supervisor insisted that I go to the military mental health office. It wasn't a suggestion.

* * *

Over the next couple months leading up to my move to Ottawa, I was diagnosed with obsessive-compulsive personality disorder and major depressive disorder. I started talking to a therapist regularly, went on medication to help me sleep and to level out my serotonin levels. I was skeptical at first, and I tried to dart out the door of the clinic without being seen. After a few sessions, the stigma eased, and I felt more comfortable. It had been more than a decade since my last head injury, so it never clicked for me at the time where all of my issues could be traced back.

The whole concept of therapy was completely foreign to me. I hated talking about myself, only my siblings understood what our family life was like, and I had trouble dropping the facade of everything being A-OK. Therapy is hard, there are no two ways about it. A mental health professional is trained to take you out of your comfort zone in order to get you to see where and how you can help yourself. These sessions were the first time I ever spoke to anyone about my dad and our messed up relationship. I always thought that I was who I was despite my upbringing rather than because of it. That realization really affected me. The need to control my environment and to be perfect actually stemmed from somewhere concrete. There were reasons why I desperately craved being *good enough* for everyone around me, but never felt like I could live up to my own expectations of what that looked like.

My therapist and I worked on ways that I could develop the skills I needed to say "no" to things that were going to overwhelm me, and to focus on doing well at what was already on my plate. We addressed the solely negative feedback that I would give myself in order to propel myself to excellence; we worked to change the narrative that ran through my head. Therapy made sense. Now, common, rational sense would dictate that I would take these amazing lessons and newfound understanding forward into my everyday life, and I did work hard at it for a while, but ultimately my contorted instincts took over as my environment changed with the new posting. Perhaps if there was some sort of stability in my life at that time, I could have broken the pattern, but I'll never know.

I moved to Ottawa in October of 2013, I still had a way to go to finish my doctorate and now I would start a new full-time job, in a new organization, and have limited time to work on it. True to form, moving to Ottawa was not a solution, instead it was the catalyst for starting my toxic cycle over again. I was quickly integrated into my new unit, and I was assigned a monumental workload. My employment record preceded me; I came action-packed to my new unit with a reputation for being able to take on a lot. In addition to my more-than-full-time job, I was still trying to work on my post-graduate degree, and I took on teaching at the training school that was affiliated with my new unit, as well as delivering a course at RMC.

I became extremely engrossed and personally invested in one of the projects that was assigned to me. Much like at the research centre, the people working on the project were experts in their fields; what we were working on was going to revolutionize the way business was done in active military environments. I quickly became a go-to resource for many in this segment of the military community. I traveled all over the world participating in conferences, field exercises, and training courses. I was out of the office and out of the country more than I was in. Sometimes, I didn't know what time zone I was in from one day to the next. I loved every second, but the things I had valued in the past started to fall off the rails again—my doctorate.

Despite my personal failings, I had led a pretty charmed career to this point. I was still fairly gung-ho about being in the military and I was proud of my service. Ottawa, unfortunately, changed all of that for me. Maybe I was becoming less tolerant of the authoritarian nature of the military? Typically, a posting to Ottawa is an endpoint for many officers in their careers. Ottawa is filled to the brim with officers from different elements (Army, Navy, Air Force, and Special Forces), with varying career experience and it has a top-heavy hierarchy with a disproportionate number of *big wigs* all in the same place. Being a major in a field unit carries some weight, but majors in Ottawa are a dime a dozen and we're basically cannon fodder. It is a dog-eat-dog world.

I have developed this notion that there are three types of officers in Ottawa. First, Officer Type One: those who were like me, who wanted to do well, but not at the expense of quality or safety of the troops who their project(s) affected. Second, Officer Type Two: those who are serving their remaining contract time in a cushy office job waiting to retire with their pension in hand. Finally, Officer Type Three: those officers whose only goal in life is to advance through the ranks, at any cost and often at the expense of officer types one and two. In my first job in Ottawa, I was officer type one who was being led by an officer type three. I wasn't willing to sacrifice my integrity or the validity of my project to boost his profile. Our relationship imploded like a sinking submarine in the Marianas Trench. By Christmas of 2015, I found myself *fired* from a job I had become emotionally attached to, and again, needed to work with my career manager to find myself other military employment. I came to realize that very few of the qualities I thought made a good officer were actually valued in the Ottawa military environment—honesty, integrity, accountability, standing up for your troops, and creativity or innovation. Enter meltdown number two, stage left. I had just turned thirty-five and felt like I was going through a midlife crisis.

* * *

The one redeeming factor about moving to Ottawa, was meeting my husband. Had a series of events not lined up at just the right time, Steve and I would have been passing ships in the night. In reality, Steve and I had met years earlier in 2009 on a military exercise that I was invited to observe in Suffield, Alberta. He doesn't remember meeting me, and frankly, since my last concussion, I don't remember him either—a sweet reprieve for him. We crossed paths again in early 2015 when I was a course officer for a specialty course in Borden, Ontario. Steve was a student; he was on my radar to participate in a trial that I was organizing for my project the following year because he had done so well on the course. We were indirect colleagues who ended up coming together as something more, serendipitously, months later. He is my rock. Every personal quality that I lack or am weak in, he is strong. His patience is endless, he is communicative and empathetic beyond description. We are like the opposite sides of the same coin and we work almost symbiotically. Prior to meeting Steve, I had been in other relationships, but I never really needed anyone—I was extremely independent (sometimes to a fault). I wanted to need Steve and I realized that with him, needing someone didn't mean I had to sacrifice my independence.

When Steve and I started dating he lived in Trenton, Ontario and I was in Ottawa (a few hour drive apart). It was great getting to know each other with a little separation. Very early in our relationship, Steve was faced with the challenge of dealing with my yo-yoing mental health. His experience in the military was entirely different than mine. As a non-commissioned member (NCM), his roles and responsibilities were tailored to a specific environment and he excelled at both of his military occupations. As an NCM he was sheltered from a lot of the military politics and bureaucracy by his superiors; he was allowed to focus on his task and expertise without the overarching relational mind games that so many officers have to endure. Steve gave me a gift that I wasn't aware I needed, he listened to me without judgement, and he was there for me when I felt like my career and faith in the military institution was crumbling around me.

After being unceremoniously asked to leave my last job, I was posted within Ottawa into a new unit within the same building. For the fourth time in my career, I was in a position that was not designated for my military occupation, but this time I was working in a completely unfamiliar environment. Through this posting, I came to understand that I am resilient in the face of the occupational unknown. I have a set of basic skills and experience that allowed me to mold myself into the required role, which was forward thinking and responsive to the integration of new hi-tech equipment in a military environment. As an engineer, with project management and planning experience, I found that I could take a strategic outlook on issues that could be solved with the application of existing or experimental technology. I was quite surprised that I could assimilate so quickly into my new role in this unit.

This was also the first time that I had a female boss. She was a civilian, with no military experience, but she had worked with the Department of National Defence (DND) since her early twenties. She understood the bureaucracy within the Ottawa military environment and had empathy for what had happened to me in my last job. During the first six months of that job posting, I felt heard, valued, and understood. My boss also appreciated that I was still trying to better myself academically and we both tried hard to accommodate my studies into my schedule. Things seemed to go well, my job was interesting, and I was given a lot more autonomy to carry out my responsibilities without having to ask for permission first. I felt trusted. Steve began the process of retiring (due to a medical condition) from the military in late 2016, and he moved to Ottawa to be with me. Eighteen years into serving in the military and it finally felt like most aspects of my life were starting to line up the way I had expected them too. Don't hold your breath though . . .

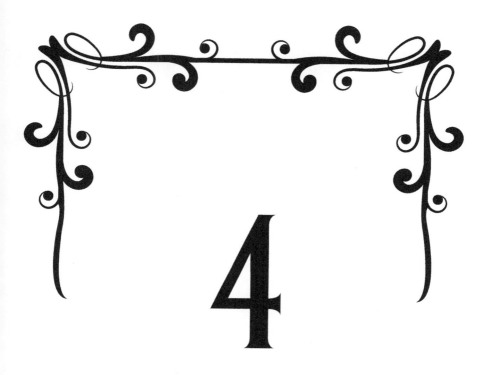

4

Flipping a Switch

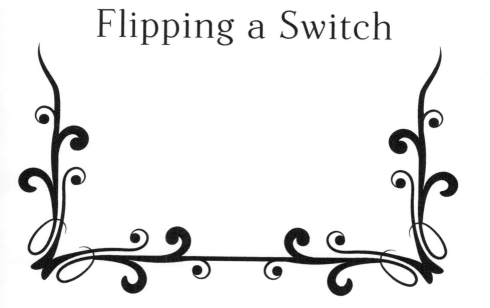

On the afternoon of December 16, 2016, my life changed forever.

One of the perks of my new job was that I was tasked to attend quite a few military technology symposiums. Some were held in really fun places, like Orlando, Florida. Steve decided to accompany me on this particular trip, so we could see the sights and go to the amusement parks after my meetings were over each day; it was going to be a really fun trip.

Steve and I were scheduled to fly home from Orlando, via Montreal, very late in the evening on December 16. My meetings had ended at around noon that day, so we decided to spend the afternoon at a theme park enjoying the beautiful weather before we hopped on a plane back to sub-zero Canada. I love theme parks, I always have. My maternal grandparents had been snowbirds when I was growing up, becoming temporary transplants into the Gulf Coast climate of Florida, so they could avoid Canadian winters. We visited several times and my Poppa was not one to miss out on the opportunity to take his grandkids to theme parks. Steve and I opted to go to my favorite Florida theme park as it had all the scariest rides, the best junk food, and the most interesting attractions. I wanted to show Steve why I loved this park so much!

The weather was gorgeous. I had a path that I liked to take around the park, which lead us to the scariest roller coasters first while our stomachs were still empty, and then eventually steered us into the direction of the water-rides, almost at the end of the day—no one likes to walk around, stand in line, or ride in wet clothing. I had a tried and true system for enjoying this theme park. All of the adventure went off without a hitch, we were having an amazing time, and enjoyed more than our fair share of theme park snacks, until after the water-rides . . .

There are three main attractions after the water-rides, all of them are high energy and adrenaline filled, with absorbing storylines and are a feast for your senses. We were soaking wet, a little bit chilled, and slightly in a rush to catch our plane, but we decided that we wanted to finish the park out properly without wasting any time. I had read that they had changed the profile of the last roller coaster we planned to ride by adding new sections of the track, and had augmented the storyline you enjoy as you're waiting in line—I was super excited to try it out! This ride is insane and there are some things you should know; it reaches a maximum speed of just under 110 km/h and has *seven* inversions throughout the course; the gravitational force equivalent (G-force) experienced by a rider is calculated to be four times standard gravity (39.2 m/s^2); it is a vicious ride that tests your intestinal fortitude; and all riders have to go through a security check and metal detectors before they get on the ride to prevent falling objects from potentially impaling unsuspecting victims when they come out of one of the loops. It's one of my absolute favorites.

We waited in line and even stood around for an extra six or seven cycles, so we could sit in the front row; it was going to be our last ride before leaving and I was hyper with anticipation. In this ride you sit in a suspended seat and your feet are free to hang as you go through the experience. You have a metal, over-the-shoulders harness with tough padding around your ears that secures you into the seat, with a car-seat buckle going between your legs and latching to the harness to keep it in place. Right away, as soon as I was buckled in, something didn't feel right; I kept trying to pull the harness down one more notch so I felt more secure, but I couldn't do it. It was like it was stuck even though I had tons of room between it and my body. By then, the platform under our feet lowered and we were on our way. I started panicking almost immediately. My head and ears were being battered into the metal harness as we went through each twist and turn. At the beginning of each inversion, my wet clothes would have my body sliding up the seat until my shoulders hit the top of the harness (that was supposed to be down tighter), and then I would slam back down when the G-forces increased as you passed the top of the loop. My ears were ringing, I was feeling sick to my stomach, and my brain was reverberating repeatedly off each side of my skull. The sudden stop at the end of the ride careened my body to the top of the harness, extending my neck to its full capacity. As the ride came to a complete stop, the back of my head smashed into the left shoulder harness. I felt my brain get thrown to the front of my skull, squish like a water balloon, and then ricochet back to its neutral position. Everything went black.

By the time the ride stopped at its passenger off-load position, I had come to again—nothing felt right—I was cold, clammy, sheet white, and very weak. Steve needed to help me off the ride. At the time, he was super amped up and he didn't really notice that I wasn't right until we were ushered off the ride and were standing at the top of the first set of stairs back down to the ground floor. I was so dizzy, I needed to sit down. I didn't know exactly what had happened before the blackout; I couldn't explain it to Steve; I was having difficulty finding the words.

It was months before I could remember the exact feelings and sensations of the disastrous ride. I must have recovered my physical bearings enough to walk out of the park with Steve, and to seem like I was a functioning human being, but I don't remember. We boarded the plane and went home a few hours later. Steve told me later that the plane ride wasn't good for me; I would normally pass out, dead asleep on a plane (which for an insomniac like myself, is a great achievement and I always look forward to it), but that trip was different. Apparently, I asked Steve for pain-killers for a persistent headache several times, not having remembered that I'd already taken the maximum dose right after the plane disembarked from the gate. I was restless and my temperature was fluctuating—hot, then cold, then back again. I was acting claustrophobic and panicked.

Getting to Ottawa was a great relief, I thought everything would be better. Here is where my ability to make decisions reached an all time low; I opted not to seek medical attention once I was back in Canada. I could blame my poor decision-making or my newly acquired brain injury, but there were other factors that definitely influenced the decision not to go to the hospital. It was the start of Christmas vacation; Steve and I were going to be back on a plane in four days' time to fly to Alberta to visit friends, and then drive to the Rockies to go skiing. It was going to be Steve's and my first real vacation that didn't involve camping, and I didn't want to put a damper on our plans. Anyways, I felt that I'd recovered fairly quickly from brain shakes before, so why would this one be any different? Also, the military medical facility was going to be closed or with minimum staff for the Christmas break. I would have had to go to the civilian emergency room; I felt that my injury didn't warrant the time and would be a waste of resources during a busy season. I promised both Steve and myself that I would go to the doctor as soon as Christmas vacation was over, even just to document the injury because technically, I had been on a work trip when it occurred.

I spent the next couple of days resting and slowly packing for the trip out West, nothing felt right though. The cognitive symptoms of a brain injury were in full swing; I was very slow processing information that was spoken to me; it felt like I was only hearing half of what was said because I would be busy dealing with the initial information and could not catch the backend of it; I couldn't focus on reading or TV, words looked like they were doubled horizontally, and I couldn't keep track of images on the screen; and my difficulty with word-finding continued, and it was incredibly difficult for others to carry out a conversation with me.

Physically, I definitely had whiplash as my neck was agonizing and tight, I thought my skull was going to snap off if I moved too quickly in one direction or another. Bright lights and loud noises were excruciating for my persistent headache. The pain in my neck seemed to extend like a rooted tree branch through my thoracic and lumbar spine; sitting or standing too long was out of the question. If I stood up too fast, dizziness and unstable blood pressure would force me to sit down. Nausea was ever-present; I spent quite a bit of the next couple days lying in bed not sleeping, in a chemically induced cloud of over-the-counter muscle relaxants and painkillers. I was exhausted.

By the time the Alberta trip came around, I had the dizziness under control and had learned to manage my ongoing headache; it was now a dull ache in my brain rather than a battering ram at both the front and back. I felt like I was on the mend, like there was no problem. The plane ride, again, felt like my senses were being abused and my skull was being squeezed, but it was marginally better than the trip home from Florida. I believe that both Steve and I were being overly optimistic about my condition because we wanted this trip to be amazing; Steve was going to meet my best friend, Beverly, for the first time and he was going to learn to ski! I really wanted both of those things for him.

When Bev saw me, she immediately knew that something wasn't right. I wasn't my quick-witted, pithy self; I was slow to respond during conversation and wasn't gung-ho to go on city adventures. Bev and I met in 2006, a few months before she turned forty, at the Ottawa marathon race weekend. She had a goal to qualify for the Boston marathon—she did it! Bev is a Canadian Forces veteran, a military wife, a mother, a teacher, a runner, a cross fit beast, and the best friend anyone could ask for. We quickly bonded over our collective cynicism for humanity and realized that we were kindred spirits because of random, common experiences. We might go months without talking to each other, but we understand that we're both busy and can pick up exactly where we left off the next time we see each other. Bev subscribes to the premise of sustained honesty, if she sees something she doesn't like, she's going to speak up—she saw something happening to me during that trip that she didn't like. She also made me promise that I would see a doctor when I got back. Bev told Steve, under no uncertain terms, that he was charged with taking care of me, otherwise he'd have to answer to her.

After the visit with Bev, we drove to the Rockies for Christmas and our ski vacation. Having grown up in Alberta, I have been downhill skiing since I was very young; it was another one of those activities that Dad and I had competed in: who could go the fastest, challenge each other to go on the hardest runs, go off the beaten path between runs through skinny tree trails, etc. I was a pretty good skier, but I had learned to hate it because of how stressful of an activity it had become during my childhood. This was supposed to be an opportunity for me to take the sport back as my own. We were in Fairmont, BC, which is where I learned to ski as a kid. Steve had never skied before, so I wanted him to have a lesson before I took him on an easy chair run. We started on the bunny hill, so I could show Steve how to snowplough, turn, and use his poles (the basics before his lesson). We were going down the hill so slowly, stopping every few turns to assess, or because Steve would end up on his butt. It was pretty fun! While Steve was in class, I decided to get a few runs in on my own.

I knew this hill inside and out, so I figured that I'd take it easy, relax on the chairlift, and try to enjoy the sport I had grown to despise. The chairlift is where my undiagnosed post-concussion symptoms started to flare up worse than the uncomfortable baseline that I'd grown accustomed to over the last week. I was on the chair by myself, and I started to feel very light-headed as the chair progressed up the hill; I began sweating profusely (even though it was below -20°C), and my head was pounding; the 300-metre elevation change from the start of the chair ride to the end was very scary. I was able to get myself together enough to disembark from the chair safely at the top, but immediately had to sit down to gather myself. I could feel that I had sweat through my parka and started shivering uncontrollably. There were only two ways down; I ski down or I talk to a ski patrol folk to let them know there was a problem. I seriously contemplated the second option, but my ego got in the way.

I started down the hill very slowly. My peripheral vision was playing tricks on me; I got scared every time another skier would head in my direction, I thought they were going to hit me. After travelling about fifty metres down the hill, I had to take a break. My muscles felt like jelly and my joints were aching from the effort. I was freezing, my head was pounding, and it was going to take me forever to get down the hill. I made the executive decision to get down as quickly as I could, but any time I started to pick up speed, my vision would grey out at the edges and it would start tunneling—this effect would dissipate as soon as I stopped and stood still. About halfway down the hill I had to stop and vomit in the treeline. I made it down eventually, but it took me just under an hour, Steve was finishing his lesson. Needless to say, that was my last run. Steve was perfectly content spending another hour on the bunny hill, while I rested and dried out in the chalet; my entire body was soaked in sweat from top to bottom. Concerned about my condition, we decided that we were done skiing for the week, and we'd spend the rest of the time relaxing and going to the hot springs.

When we returned to Ottawa, I had to go back to work almost immediately and Steve was starting his first semester of vocational rehabilitation training, taking the computer systems technician course at Algonquin College. Over the remaining vacation period, the relaxation time had really helped. Despite the promises that I had made to Steve, Bev, and myself, I didn't go seek medical attention right away because my headache had been knocked back to a dull roar, and physically, I was feeling better. I felt that I had some critical, self-imposed deadlines at work that needed to take priority.

I never told anyone at work that there was something going on.

I returned to work in a cubicle environment. Being surrounded by bright fluorescent lights, computer screens, and the hum of day-to-day conversation that were incredibly distressing and disorienting. Sitting in the standard issue, plastic, "ergonomic" office chair, was wreaking havoc on my back and neck. It was torture. I started to spend more and more time away from my desk, trying to find quiet, darker spaces where I could work with pen and paper to do rough drafts of my project deliverables. I felt overwhelmed by the amount of work I had to do, but also by the social requirements of working in a close-space office environment. I felt dumber, legitimately dumber. I couldn't access knowledge that I knew had been previously stored in my brain. I had difficulties with word recall and would get lost in the middle of a sentence, sometimes changing subjects because I forgot what I was talking about, or other times getting frustrated with myself because I couldn't remember a simple word. I once sat at my desk, completely distracted from what I was supposed to be doing because I couldn't remember why we use the word "the" or what its purpose was in a sentence.

I started to isolate myself from everyone, including my boss. I never let her know I was struggling until it became readily apparent that I was going to miss every single one of my deadlines. Prior to my injury, my boss was really impressed with the level and quality of the deliverables that I would churn out. My work had elevated the status of our two-person section, and she was really pleased with my work ethic and efficiency. After my injury, my productivity was reduced to a trickle and I found myself spending longer and longer hours at the office, preferring to work when no one else was there, but also to put in the extra hours that I needed to equal a function of 50 percent pre-injury level.

I wasn't sleeping at night, I was in pain, and consumed by the stress of going to work the next day. My relationship with Steve was strained because I was frustrated all the time with everything around me. The trust that my boss had in my work gradually started to degrade and our personal interactions became more infrequent and quite curt. I don't know what she thought was going on with me. Perhaps she thought that I was gearing up to retire from the military and that I intended just to coast out the rest of my contract in officer type two style? She didn't ask any questions. I think she had seen that happen before with a previous employee, so she just chalked it up to institutional fatigue. I also started to notice how much she had relied on my work to maintain her own prominence in the unit. When I didn't complete things by the deadline that I had assigned myself and had previously communicated with her, she would get frustrated with me and snippy with her responses.

My social life was also suffering. I've always been an introvert who could temporarily pretend to be an extrovert for limited periods of time when the situation called for it. Post-concussion, I became the queen of making plans and then canceling on the day of the event. It was difficult to talk to me because I was still having issues focusing on conversations and paying attention to what people were actually saying; there was a lot of unconscious head nodding, "yes"-ing and "no"-ing where I thought it was appropriate; I rarely caught enough of the discussion to contribute to it. I was so trapped in my head that I couldn't actively start a conversation on my own, except to point out things that I might need. When I wasn't at work putting in long hours, I spent a lot of time in bed, not sleeping, but trying to find a comfortable position while being in the dark and quiet.

Acknowledging that I needed help was quite possibly the most difficult task in my recovery. It took almost four months before I accepted how much the roller coaster accident had affected me cognitively, physically, and mentally. By then, the symptoms of post-concussion syndrome had already settled in for the long haul. For the next couple months, I was subjected to a battery of tests, x-rays, MRIs, and physiotherapy. I still tried to work full-time, carrying the same workload while adding in these medical appointments. My medical practitioners all concluded that I was suffering the aftermath of a severe concussion. I wasn't severely physically impaired, and despite my seeming loss of brain function, I still scored above average on the neuropsychological exams, they told me that there was little they could do. I had four MRIs on my brain, lumbar spine, thoracic spine, and cervical spine. Aside from cervical spasming, nothing of note was documented from that imagery. I was told that neuroplasticity, or the brain's ability to rewire itself, will take time and that I needed to be patient.

THE TRUTH ABOUT CONCUSSIONS

A concussion, also known as mild traumatic brain injury, or mTBI, has a series of classic symptoms, but not every brain injured person experiences all of them. There may not be any physical evidence of the brain injury that will show up in standard CT and MRI imagery. We, as an advanced society, just don't know enough about this organ to be able to chart all of the nuances associated with a brain that isn't functioning properly.

A concussion is a cumulative change in neurological function as a result of a bump, blow, or jolt to the head. The most concrete way to describe what an mTBI is, is to examine the mechanism of action. The bump, blow, or jolt received will result in the violent movement of the brain within the skull. This sudden movement will cause a dysregulation in the release of the chemical neurotransmitters, glutamate, and γ-aminobutyric acid (GABA), which throw the brain's ability to signal out of sync. Glutamate is the brain's main excitatory neurotransmitter, and GABA is the primary inhibitory neurotransmitter. The balance of these two neurochemicals in the brain is crucial for normal neurological function. The violent action associated with a mTBI can also result in the swelling of brain tissue, which can reduce the flow of oxygen and glucose via the blood, which essentially starves the brain cells.[6]

The symptoms in sport-related concussions are typically overcome within seven to ten days. That symptom recovery time increases to within three months for non-athletes.[7] Unfortunately, approximately 33% of patients will have continued symptoms after the three month mark. Of that 33% of patients, 30% will have persistence of at least three of the classic post-concussion syndrome criteria symptoms six months post-injury.[8] The classic post-concussion syndrome criteria symptoms are headache, dizziness, fatigue, irritability, insomnia, difficulty in concentration or memory, and intolerance of stress, both physical and emotional.[9] In 2017, a review of long-term post-concussion data found that only 27% of patients who still met the post-concussion syndrome criteria three months after their injury eventually made a full recovery.[10] If we assume that there are one thousand patients who have a concussion; at the three month mark, 330 of those patients will still be experiencing post-concussion symptoms; of those 330 patients, only 89 of them will recover fully, leaving 241 with persistent long-term symptoms!

If you are one of the lucky ones who does recover and walk away without persistent symptoms following a mTBI, you aren't off scot-free. You will always be more susceptible to repeat concussions than someone who has never had one, particularly during the first year after the initial brain injury. A second concussion while you're still in "recovery mode" could occur with less force than the first injury, and will more likely take longer to recover from.[11]

The consequences of brain injuries have dominated the news media during the twenty-first century. The national football and hockey leagues have commissioned research and large-scale patient studies within their own populations. Game rules and protective equipment regulations have been changed in an effort to quell the number of concussion occurrences. Unlike other organs in the body, it isn't quite as simple to biopsy brain tissue to check for injury without potentially having large scale consequences for other physical, cognitive or executive functions down the line. In addition, no brain is wired exactly the same way; because of this, former and current players are being compelled to "will their brains" to science upon the event of their death. One progressive and degenerative brain disorder they are trying to understand is chronic traumatic encephalopathy (CTE). The physical signs of CTE, at this time, can only be documented post-mortem.[12] Post-mortem social studies, in coordination with brain histological work, have linked CTE to dementia and progressive loss of executive function, memory, and mood instability. Over time, these symptoms can lead to risk-taking or suicidal behaviors. CTE isn't the only potential long-term issue for someone who has had repeated concussions.[13] Patients may also have an increased risk for Parkinson's disease and depression, later in life.[14] So far, the populations used within these studies are primarily men, and almost exclusively, professional athletes.[15] Where does this leave the rest of us mere mortals?

Concussions are a common injury, however, Canadians as a whole have very limited knowledge on what a concussion is, how a concussion should be treated, or the resources that are available to them.[16] In Canada, in 2016 to 2017, more than 46,000 concussions were diagnosed in youth aged five to nineteen years old. Male patients accounted for approximately 26,000 of the reported diagnoses, with 54% being attributed to sports and recreation, the other 46% were caused by assaults or self-harm, and other unintentional causes (ex. bike, car accident, or fall). The remaining diagnoses were for female patients, with 45% being caused by sports and recreation, and a higher proportion attributed to assaults or self-harm, and other unintentional causes.[17] These numbers are staggering!

In 2016, *The Canadian Journal of Neurological Sciences* published a study estimating that the international, pooled incident rate of concussion for all ages is approximately 3.5 per 1000 people per year.[18] Statistically more men are affected by concussions annually, however, there is a growing body of evidence that suggests women take longer to recover from concussions, have more severe symptoms, and are physically more at risk of getting concussions than men.[19]

FACT: WOMEN ARE PHYSIOLOGICALLY DIFFERENT FROM MEN.

Traumatic brain injuries, including concussions, or mild TBIs, affect women differently. At Michigan State University, Dr. Travey Covassin (a Canadian by birth) carries out epidemiological studies focusing on concussions in female athletes. Her research indicates that not only do women experience more severe symptoms than men, but they take longer to recover.[20] While men typically recover from the most severe symptoms of a concussion within ten to fourteen days, women take longer to see the same neurocognitive improvements, sometimes up to four weeks; lingering impairments were generally related to memory and concentration. Dr. Covassin attributes these differences in the rate of recovery to anatomical differences between the male and female brains. Nerve impulses within the male brain are faster compared to those in the female brain. It is postulated that this difference in communication speed could result in a faster healing process post-concussion for men.[21]

Everything considered, all sports and their increased capacity for risk-taking behaviors, men account for the majority of concussions. That being said though, when comparing similar activities or sports that have the same rules for both men and women (ex. basketball or soccer), the rate of concussions in women is twice as high as for men.[22] Again, anatomical differences could be at play here. In soccer, as an example, heading the ball results in a greater transmission of force through the female brain and cervical spine because of the greater "ball-to-head size ratio."[23] Women have smaller surface areas on their forehead to absorb the resulting impact. This concept can easily be extended to other causal impact types and neuroanatomical areas of impact.

A study published in *Medicine and Science in Sports and Exercise* in 2005 found that the "head-neck angular acceleration" experienced by women when receiving a blow to the head is significantly greater than that experienced by men. This biomechanical measurement of angular acceleration between the head and neck takes into account both the force of the impact to the head and the displacement of the head caused by the impact.[24] The gender difference can be explained by examining the differences in cervical musculature. Women are less likely to be as heavily muscled in the shoulder and neck area as compared to men. Our anatomical center of gravity is lower, lending women to be proportionally sturdier in the lumbar and hip region. This difference in musculature means that, in general, women have less ability to absorb the angular acceleration associated with a head impact, resulting in a higher rate of concussions when comparing the same injury mechanism.

The female hormone cycle may also affect the recovery and achievable outcomes following concussion. In 2014, a study was published in *The Journal of Head Trauma Rehabilitation* by Dr. Jeffrey Bazarian, from the University of Rochester Medical Center, concluded that hormonal changes of progesterone and estrogen during a woman's menstrual cycle can have a negative effect on the symptoms experienced post-concussion.[25] The researchers found that women who experienced head trauma during the last two weeks of their menstrual cycle (the luteal phase, when progesterone is at its highest level) were at higher risk of experiencing worse post-concussion symptoms compared to those who were injured during the first two weeks of their cycle (the follicular phase), or those women who use the contraceptive pill or other forms of pharmaceutical birth control. The hormone progesterone is proven to have a calming effect and can improve a woman's cognition, memory, and mood.[26] Researchers followed the recovery process of women over the course of their post-concussion rehabilitation and found that progesterone levels in women who received a head injury during the luteal phase declined overall following their head trauma. It is theorized that sustaining a head injury during the luteal phase results in a slowing of progesterone production. This creates a "withdrawal effect" making the post-concussion symptoms such as headache, dizziness, and nausea worse.[27] The sudden drop in progesterone levels renders the symptoms of a concussion more severe.

Dr. Angela Colantonio, the director of the Rehabilitation Sciences Institute at the University of Toronto, presented a study in *The Journal of Women's Health* in 2010, which tracked the outcomes of 104 women who had experienced a TBI with respect to their menstrual cycles, fertility, and pregnancies.[28] Researchers found that 68% of the study participants had irregular periods following their injury and they also reported higher incidences of reduced mental health and cognitive function.[29] More research is required to understand the exact neuroanatomical reason for fluctuations in hormonal levels post-concussion.

Overall, women are more likely to report their symptoms to healthcare practitioners than men are, however they are less likely to seek out specialized treatment.[30] In athletics, men are more likely to hide their symptoms in order to not be seen as being somehow inferior or not wanting to let down their coach or teammates. Due to the prevalence, prestige, and accessibility of male professional sports teams, men are more likely to have an opportunity to "go pro" and don't want to sacrifice their career for a head injury.[31] There is less of an opportunity for women to play professional sports, and even if they do, there is no money in it, so the notion of a woman not reporting a head injury to avoid sacrificing a potential career is far less common.

Interestingly, women are less likely to report concussions that aren't sports-related, those that occur during day-to-day activity, instead, they simply get on with their day.[32] Katherine Snedaker, the founder of the non-profit group Pink Concussions, believes that gender bias with respect to healthcare is partially to blame for the lower reporting incidents of non-sports-related concussions.[33] She points to studies that have found that women's pain is often being discounted when related to mental and physical injuries, as women are less likely to be prescribed painkillers in hospital than men, despite reporting higher levels of pain. A 2008 study of American patients undergoing cardiac surgery, for instance, found that women were more likely to be given sedatives than men, who were more likely to be given painkillers—perhaps because doctors implicitly assume that women's distress is more emotional than physiological. Another study found that women reporting to the emergency room with acute abdominal pain were less likely to be prescribed painkillers than men with the same complaint.[34] These incidents of gender bias in the healthcare community are indicative that women's health concerns, collectively, need to be taken more seriously. Gone are the times when you can explain women's pain away as they're "just suffering from the vapors."

FACT: MOST RESEARCH AND LITERATURE ON MTBIS IS BASED ON MALE SUBJECTS.

Gender issues with respect to concussions, their symptoms and their projected recovery outcomes are an understudied topic.[35] Most of the research that exists consists of studies of male subjects who play professional or high-level sports, particularly in male-dominated, full contact team environments (football, hockey, rugby, etc.). Because most of the studies available on brain trauma use male subjects, treatment protocols, diagnoses practices, clinicians' knowledge, and even the expectations that the female patient, their guardian(s), and coaches have are often misguided.

MY POST-CONCUSSION EXPERIENCE

There are entire books published on the classic signs and symptoms of initial mTBI and the consequential post-concussion syndrome. I can only speak about the physical, cognitive, and emotional symptoms that I experienced personally.

I suppose the first thing that was outwardly noticeable following my concussion was my inability to walk in a straight line. It wasn't just the initial dizziness, but rather a complete unawareness of where my body was in space. Proprioception is known as the sixth sense, it is like your internal gyroscope, and it is the link between your brain and where your body parts are located in space. Proprioception is mediated by proprioceptive neurons located within muscles, tendons, and joints.[36] The central nervous system links feedback from these neurons with information from the vision and vestibular systems in order to create a "sense" of your body position, how it's moving, and the acceleration of your movements through space. After my concussion, I experienced changes in my vision and vestibular systems that negatively impacted my proprioceptive capability, which I will talk about shortly. In addition, I kept overreaching when I was walking, I couldn't grab things with my hands on the first try, and I fell and wobbled a lot. Glassware was not safe in my vicinity. Physiotherapy and occupational therapy were important in helping me relearn and readjust to my new normal in terms of body movement.

As I demonstrated previously, my ability to focus and concentrate while I was at work was severely inhibited by a combination of light and sound hypersensitivity with a chronic headache. When I was in the office, I felt like there was a constant hum of sound, like many people speaking at the same time, but I couldn't understand what they were saying. On more than one occasion I was startled when someone entered my cubicle while my back was to the opening and they started to talk to me. Their speaking blended in with all of the surrounding commotion, and I didn't actually know they were there until they tapped me on the shoulder. Being startled feels different when your brain doesn't know how to resolve the fight or flight response. I am not a screamer or a jumper when I'm scared. I'm not the person who will immediately respond to danger the way normal people do. I have to process what is going on for a fraction of a second before I can make a decision about what to do. Steve and I used to joke that I was the person you wanted to be with if you stumbled across a bear in a forest. Most people would reactively run, I have to contemplate my options before my flight instinct kicks in. Bear breakfast. I've always been like that, but now with the brain impairment, when I was startled, I couldn't take that second to calm down the neurotransmitters that were firing in my body telling me to do something to react. Instead, my body would respond by initiating a panic attack. So, not only was I slow to react, I also now reacted completely inappropriately to perceived danger. Bear breakfast, with a side of ill-timed anxiety—tasty. People learned quite quickly not to sneak up on me.

My vision was also dramatically impacted. My ability to eye track from left to right wasn't badly affected, but looking up and down (without moving my head) would make my mind spin. In addition, when I was presented with text on a screen or a page, the words would be doubled horizontally and slightly out of alignment to the left. This diplopia is a very common complaint following a concussion; It is caused by the alignment of your eyes diverging in different directions as you try to focus on an object in the near frame. It can be the result of damage to the muscles or nerves around the eyes during the impact, but can also be attributed to lingering frontal lobe damage. I was very lucky to have found an optometrist who had just attended a workshop on post-concussion ocular symptoms. She was able to quickly tweak my diplopia issues by adjusting the prescription of my glasses and adding a differential prism in each lens to accommodate my eye alignment issues. This small but significant change restored my depth perception and re-established some of my proprioceptive ability while wearing glasses. I was ecstatic!

I have also experienced the loss of some of my peripheral vision in my right eye. Despite seeing two different optometrists and a neuro-ophthalmologist, as well as doing three different field of view tests to confirm the issue, I still have yet to receive a diagnosis or explanation for this deficit. The combination of photophobia (sensitivity to light) and my loss in peripheral vision makes driving at night near impossible. I've become a "day-walker" and I rarely go out at night anymore, unless my husband can drive me.

One of the most disturbing symptoms that I still experience is difficulty understanding a one-on-one conversation unless I'm looking directly at the person. Also, if there is an excessive amount of environmental noise or multiple people speaking at the same time, I can't understand a single word anyone is saying. This is the symptom that affected me the most while I was working in the cubicle environment. I had multiple hearing tests and the results were perfect every time; the tests didn't even register any of the normal loss in frequency range associated with aging. I was also referred to an ear, nose, and throat specialist. Unfortunately, he couldn't diagnose a specific injury either. It wasn't until I started reading papers and doing my own research online that

I learned about Auditory Processing Disorder (APD) and its prevalence following repeated concussive injuries. I postulated the theory to my medical officer, and he agreed to send me to a neuro-audiologist. The hearing tests that are done on those for APD are not the same as regular tests. The testing focuses on not only how well you hear sound, but how well you understand the sounds that are being emitted. I was diagnosed with APD and hyperacusis (sensitivity to loud noise—in my case, in the upper frequency range). The majority of the issues that I demonstrated, with respect to understanding words and sentences, occurred when the sound was focused on my right side. If you'll recall, I also have a deficit in my field of view on my right side. My neuro-audiologist presented a theory as to why my vision and hearing on the right side were the most affected by my injury. She suggested that auditory processing requires communication between both the left and right hemispheres of the brain and the neurons that interconnect these hemispheres may have somehow been impaired in the accident, hence the directional difference in my hearing. The neuro-audiologist also explained the concept of neuroplasticity, which is the brain's ability to continually change and overcome dysfunction over time, even months or years after an injury. As an example, if a patient has sustained a mTBI that results in the loss of a specific function, the brain activity associated with that function can be transferred or reassigned to a different part of the brain through the process of synaptic remapping.[37] The concept of neuroplasticity gave me hope that many of my lingering symptoms may eventually go away over the long term. In the meantime, I could accommodate the APD by using an FM radio listening system in group environments, which amplifies a speaker's voice using a microphone and transmitting it directly to a headset or hearing aids. I am also able to cancel out background noise if it is too overwhelming. I have had to relearn how to recognize social cues that indicate when a person is going to initiate conversation. I took the ability to distinguish social cues and physical nuances for granted prior to my injury. I have also become fairly adept at reading lips to assist in my comprehension when someone is speaking to me.

Headaches are still a constant nuisance. I experience three types of headaches on a regular basis. The first type are cluster headaches that are usually focused above my right eye. These headaches are the most tolerable, shortest in duration, and they are quite easy to treat with over-the-counter painkillers. The second type of headache I experience, and also the most frequently occuring, is a cervicogenic headache. Cervicogenic headaches are considered to be secondary headaches because they are the result of another illness or physical issue.[38] In my case, they are caused by neck tension due to the whiplash I suffered during the accident. A cervical MRI showed signs that my neck was constantly spasming, and as a consequence, it stays in a very straight position, which causes strain on the cervical and occipital muscles. The third, and subsequently worst, type of headache that I suffer from are migraines. My migraines can be caused by even the slightest change in barometric pressure. I am basically a human barometer and you can predict the weather based on my head and bodily pain patterns. Migraines are absolutely crippling and they take me out of service for days at a time, the winter being particularly vicious due to the Canadian weather patterns. I take daily preventative pharmaceuticals in order to thwart their onset, but the dosage that I'm comfortable taking is only helpful about 30-40% of the time.

As a result of the complex mechanism of action that resulted in impact injury, I suffer from chronic pain, not only in my cervical spine, but also in my thoracic and lumbar spine. No definitive injury showed up in X-rays or MRI imagery within these areas, minus typical degeneration attributed to aging. This was incredibly frustrating for me because I don't have a concrete diagnosis that I can identify and blame for being in so much pain. Some days, I struggle to sit or stand for longer than five minutes, while other days my pain decreases with sustained activity. It is so counter-intuitive! It is this type of invisible injury that I was most fearful of due to the potential negative perception of the "realness" of it and the inevitable disdain from my colleagues. My biggest fear was being called a malingerer who was just trying to get a medical release from the military. Chronic pain is both physically and mentally debilitating. When you're stuck in bed, your brain goes to some pretty dark places.

Despite seeking medical attention four months post-injury, it took me quite a while to wrap my mind around how long rehabilitation was going to take. Once

I had engaged assistance, the military medical system was surprisingly responsive, but I think even they became disheartened and at a loss for how to help me when my rehabilitation timeline extended six months from starting therapy. I was incredibly stubborn about not wanting to quit working. I had this perverse sense of duty to the organization that warped me into thinking that going to get medical care was bad for my career. I attempted to work full-time for almost ten months post-injury. The sustained effort to engage meaningfully in the work environment, combined with my academic, familial, and social responsibilities, took a toll on my already fragile mental health. I gradually began to reduce my work hours with the hope the break would allow me to reintegrate at a later time. Unfortunately, my declining mental health forced me to quit working in May 2018, almost one and a half years post-injury. It took a team of people, including my primary physician and my husband, to convince me that stepping back from work was the right decision.

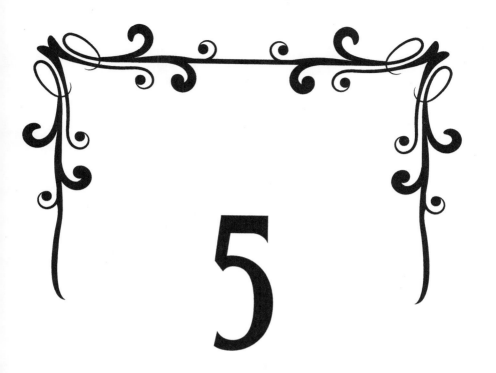

5

The Mourning After

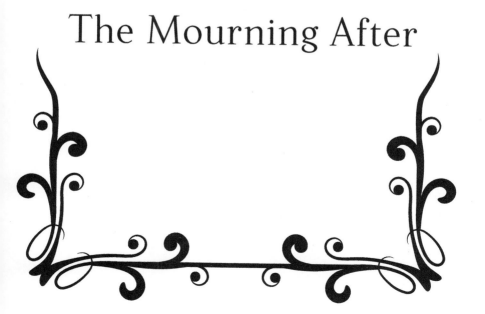

ased on the directionality of my injury, it is classed as a "coup-contrecoup."[39] This basically means that the focal point of my brain injury is two-fold. First, directly at the point of impact and also on the direct opposite side of my brain. During my accident, my brain first went forward in my skull when the roller coaster abruptly stopped, and then almost immediately slammed backwards due to an inertial effect. Because of this, I have multiple areas of my brain that are likely damaged. I say "likely" because, again, nothing showed up on the imagery that was carried out by my medical team. Multiple members of my post-concussion care team have postulated that I have injuries in my frontal lobe area as well as the amygdala; the amygdala is the primary emotional center of your brain. The combination of these focal points of damage have contributed to difficulties processing emotions (particularly anxiety, fear, and aggression), retrieving memories, and decision-making.[40]

It definitely wasn't the post-concussion physical changes that I found the most difficult to adapt to; I'd been physically injured before and can adjust my level and type of activity to accommodate. The hardest effects to handle have been, and still are, the lingering symptoms associated with executive dysfunction and loss of cognitive control. The term "executive function" is an umbrella term for the higher-level skills that a person uses to control their behaviors and general cognitive processing. In a nutshell, it is how you manage yourself in order to achieve a goal. Executive dysfunction often occurs following injury to the frontal lobe.[41]

The primary effects of executive dysfunction that I experienced following my mTBI in 2016 were:

1. Difficulties in initiating, organizing, and carrying out regular day-to-day activities;
2. An inability to think flexibly in decision-making and conversation;
3. Poor problem-solving skills;
4. An increase in impulsivity (i.e. not thinking about the consequences of my actions);
5. Mood disturbances;
6. Difficulties in social situations; and
7. Difficulties with memory, concentration, and attention.

My post-concussion mental impairment was classified as minimal loss of brain function, basically tantamount to telling me that nothing was wrong with me. I felt the medical community was saying to me, "gosh, you're lucky to have started out smarter than the average person—now, you're just like everyone else, isn't that nice?" I identified with my intelligence, memory, work ethic, efficiency, and ingenuity—now I felt like a vegetable. That dismissive diagnosis didn't sit well with me and didn't account for the loss that I was experiencing. My injury was more than invisible, I felt like I was being told it was "all in my head"—pun intended. I started questioning who I was and where I was supposed to go—*what was the point?* I didn't realize it at the time, but I was in the beginning stages of the mourning process. I was grieving.

My obsessive-compulsive traits changed post-injury. Previously, I had been obsessed with perfection and striving to constantly better myself, at the expense of my mental health. Immediately post-concussion, it felt like my perfectionism and attention to detail was going away. I was completely overwhelmed dealing with the changes to my body and brain that I didn't obsess over being fastidious. Yes, I was still concerned about disappointing people, but when it came to work deliverables, I was more concerned about not meeting deadlines instead of the quality of my work. The extra hours I was putting in at the office were just to try to maintain functionality, not to ensure I was producing a stellar product. For a brief moment in time, it was a bit liberating that I wasn't so focused on controlling everything in my wake. On several occasions, I actually said "no" to taking on more work, and I handed in first drafts rather than the finished product. My boss was having to take more responsibility for my output, and to be honest, I didn't really care. I would have NEVER said that pre-concussion.

The only real obsession that I had during my first months post-concussion was maintaining an appearance of being okay at all times. This façade and its upkeep took a toll on my physical and mental health. This is when my obsessive-compulsive characteristics started to take hold again, with a vengeance. I started to worry about everything, particularly things that weren't in my control. I worried about getting trapped in the elevator on my way up to my thirteenth floor office. I worried about being hit by cars as I crossed the road (legally). I even worried about germs and began seeking advice from "Dr. Google" for every little tingle in my throat or grumble in my stomach. I was completely overwhelmed in crowds because of the noise, but also because of the complete unpredictability of people in pack situations. One time, I went to the Rideau Mall over my lunch break to pick something up in the food court; I hadn't thought about it at the time, but it was a professional development day for schools. The mall was packed with the lunch crowd and so many teenagers. It only took one group of girls, not paying attention to where they were walking and bumping into me, as I tried to move through a corridor, for my anxiety to go through the roof! I went into a full-blown panic attack in the mall. I couldn't breathe, my chest felt so tight, I started sweating profusely, and thought I was going to pass out. I managed to make my way to the washroom into the handicapped stall where I had to lay down on the cold (and likely very dirty) tile floor to regain my sense of composure. I waited out the rest of my lunch break in the stall and then went back to work. Aside from the slight smell of pee and commercial disinfectant on my uniform, I don't think anyone noticed that I wasn't right for the rest of the day.

Panic attacks started to become a more regular occurrence, particularly when I was also dealing with one of my headaches. I became fearful about my present and future actions. I was always on edge, worried about when someone would want to have a conversation with me, worried that I wouldn't understand what they were saying, and worried that I was going to cry at work. Crying at work or showing the cracks in my composure was another no-no in my world. Ever since I was a child, showing any negative emotion aside from anger was a sign of weakness. I am, unfortunately, one of those people who cries when I'm emotionally frustrated; I've never been able to help it. I was teased mercilessly when I was a kid in school because of this peculiarity, and my dad wasn't a fan of it either. My disdain for crying in public extended into my adult life, and I worked very hard to control my emotions, so I wouldn't get to a state where crying was inevitable. The misogynistic military mentality helped reinforce the stigma around showing negative emotions in public. My brain injury seemed to completely prohibit any control over my emotional frustrations. I could always feel tension rising in my throat and it was a preemptive warning sign that my control was waning. I felt this physical alarm bell go off more and more frequently, so I would hide myself away; in my room at home, in the bathroom at work, and (on one occasion) in an electrical closet with "standing room only,", until I had myself under control. Sometimes it would take hours until I'd recovered. I was in that tiny electrical closet at work for two hours trying to breathe, stop crying, and look as if nothing had happened.

As my frustrations with my cumulative executive dysfunction mounted, I started to become very depressed. I withdrew from social interactions and my willingness to participate in group environments plummeted. My confidence was shot. My pent-up fears, anger, and frustration built up exponentially and there was no outlet or release valve for all the pressure. Prior to my injury, I would play sports, workout, or go for a run—not anymore; the symptoms of my concussion lingered and, as a result, I started to gain weight. This further contributed to my body dysmorphia—shame and embarrassment prevented me from going to the gym or for a run. I was afraid of falling off a treadmill or the side of a sidewalk because my proprioception and dizziness rendered me a huge klutz. For lack of a healthy outlet, I started to binge-watch Netflix and listen to podcasts. A lot of what I would watch and listen to would be documentaries about trauma and recovery. If staring at a TV screen was too much for me, then I would close my eyes and just listen to the commentary for hours on end. I started to disconnect from my friends and family, but I was obsessed with the recovery stories that I heard and lived vicariously through them, while not working on my own health.

One of the most interesting and fundamentally frustrating things about my brain injury was the "Good Brain Days" were scattered intermittently between all of the bad ones. On the good brain days, all of my executive functions seem to have magically righted themselves. I could think clearly, my balance was restored, I could regurgitate every word that I needed on command, and I followed conversations with little effort. However, on these days my anxiety was still present and I always felt like I was "waiting for the other shoe to drop." I was anticipating the executive dysfunction to take over and consume my life again. These good brain days were few and far between, but I couldn't relish in them because I knew it wouldn't last and I'd relapse into mTBI chaos. I had read once that good brain days will eventually string themselves together and I'd have a good brain week, and then a good brain month. At the time though, that didn't feel like part of my fore-seeable future. So, I isolated myself and wouldn't let anyone see my struggles or my successes.

When I did engage socially, I became quickly frus-trated. My mood would shift from being hopeful that I'd have a good experience to dark and brooding. I would feel the need to escape. I became ashamed to socialize with pre-injury friends, I didn't want them to see me in such a damaged state. I didn't go to my fif-teen year RMC reunion, but I was in Kingston over that weekend, and I did visit a few close friends for lunch. I just couldn't bring myself to go to the full event be-cause I didn't want people to see "how far I'd fallen." I couldn't remember faces or names of people that I had known for four years. RMC is a small school—I only graduated with 200 other people. Before my accident, I knew everyone, remembered everyone's name, the positions they held when we were at RMC and details about interactions we'd had. Not anymore. I felt like I'd be around all of these successful, high-achieving peo-ple, and I would be struggling to find words, having to explain myself. I couldn't handle it. At my ten year reunion, I had been an entirely different person; I was promoted early to major, I was working towards my doctorate, publishing scientific papers, and I had won the Teaching Excellence Award. I had nothing to show for myself this time around except a bit of brain damage and that wasn't something I was going to brag about. This was an incredibly low point for me.

At times, I would argue with people, just for the sake of arguing; I would push Steve's buttons just to get a reaction out of him. His empathy for my situation and how I was feeling started to settle on top of me like a huge weight; it felt like pity. Pity was the last thing I wanted. I tried to push him away as a distorted means of regaining some independence that I felt I had lost. That was the worst thing I could have possibly done. Steve would give me more space, but I was still hugely limited in what I could accomplish by myself. I needed him, but I didn't want to admit it. Arguing became my way of drawing him back into a conversation, rather than apologizing for my dismissive behavior. Arguing gave me a sense of power, even if my line of reasoning didn't make sense. Steve hated conflict of any type, many times he would just walk away and that would make me even angrier. To his credit, he never gave up on me. He could have easily called it quits at any time and it would have been completely understandable.

Sexual dysfunction is also quite common following head trauma. Following a head injury, your brain goes through a silent re-prioritization of where your energy can be best spent (with respect to your bodily functions) in order to optimize its recovery.[42] Breathing, vision, hearing, and digestive functions are all more important than achieving pleasure through social interaction or sex. Your sex drive is not vital to your immediate survival or recovery. Your brain essentially turns off or turns down your desire for sex as it is seen as a superfluous function. Prior to my concussion, Steve and I had a healthy sex life; after the concussion, not so much. I would attribute it partially to cognitive changes, but also because of the medication I was prescribed for pain, mental health, and muscle control. Our relationship was forced to change. If Steve would have been unwilling to adjust and work with me to accommodate my disability, our relationship would have been a secondary casualty of my accident.

Out of everyone in my family and social circle, Steve has endured the most as I've gone through the recovery process. Not only am I an almost completely different person, personality-wise than the one he fell in love with, but I'm also different in terms of how I respond to sexual stimulation. I don't like to be touched as much or the same way. My sex drive is much lower than it was previously, and even now, three years later, it still feels like I'm defective in some way. Steve is very aware of my feelings and sensitivities when it comes to sex. He works very hard to be understanding and I try very hard to understand his needs. Steve has been my rock throughout the recovery process, and he's stayed strong through this entire emotional rollercoaster. While he has definitely struggled with the changes to my personality (and sometimes inadvertently reminds me about them), he still loves me for who I have become. For him, it was probably very akin to falling in love a second time, with a different person. I look the same on the outside, but who I am has fundamentally changed. He loves me unconditionally and I believe that if the accident hadn't happened, I might have taken that for granted.

Following a brain injury, it is crucial to include a psychiatrist or a therapist in your medical team. For some reason, the medical professionals that I was dealing with were very concerned about addressing the outward physical issues associated with my accident, the painful neck and back, my vision and hearing discrepancies, and persistent headaches, but they overlooked the mental health implications of the injury. I had completed neuropsychological testing about six months after my injury because they wanted to understand how my cognitive abilities were adapting. Neuropsychological testing isn't overly useful unless there is pre-injury baseline data or if the therapist conducting the testing has a pre-existing relationship with the patient. My post-concussion neuropsychological testing showed that I performed "above average" or "superior" to the average person across the board. These results did not explain why I felt lost, like there had been a death in the family. There was a huge disconnect between who I used to be and this stranger that I became post-injury. I wasn't referred to see a therapist to talk about my loss, anger, or my feelings of isolation until almost a year after my accident.

I really lucked out when I was outsourced by the military to see a psychotherapist who specialized in recovering from trauma. Technically, he was a grief counselor. I never in a million years had considered that I was mourning my former self. My therapist and I clicked right away. We had common interests and I was really impressed with his contribution to research activities. It was easy to converse with him. He managed to help me understand that I needed a healthy outlet for all of my negative feelings, I couldn't go on yelling at Steve or watching TV all day. He was very straight talking and never made me feel like he felt sorry for me. With his help, and over many months, I managed to identify that the expectation I would regain all of my pre-injury strengths was a hindrance in my recovery, overcoming my grief, and achieving a state of acceptance. I realized I had been incredibly hard on myself, and that my inner voice was constantly telling me how useless I was, how unproductive I was, and worst of all, how stupid I had become. How I defined intelligence was entirely based on achievement and accolades. I had to acknowledge and accept the overwhelming fear of the unknown, which tormented me. My therapist allowed me the time to resolve the loss of my pre-concussion self, and he also allowed me to discover my new strengths and how to overcome my perceived weaknesses. He made me take ownership of the discovery process.

In addition to working on my positive self-image and grief counseling, I also worked with my therapist to find resources and coping mechanisms for dealing with day-to-day challenges. As an example, my memory and ability to obtain new information had been compromised, so we spent time learning tricks and tools for retaining information. To this day, these memory skills are one of the most useful everyday tools that I have in my toolbox. My mind slowly transformed from being fragmented, like a jigsaw puzzle with pieces from multiple images, to becoming more ordered again. He also helped me to re-engage with household activities; I learned to tackle cleaning and other daily chores by taking things slowly and going step-by-step. I worked within my personal boundaries; once I started something, I wasn't content until I finished it, even if I was in pain, fatigued, or struggling mentally. He knew that was a compromise I was unwilling to make, but he was happy that I was rejoining the land of the living in my own way.

My therapist recommended a very helpful book on recovering from brain injury, called *Brainlash* by Dr. Gail Denton. Through this book I learned that individuals who are very ordered and analytical in their thought processes prior to their injury can become ethically overwhelmed during their recovery.[43] I deeply identified with that sentiment. Being ethically overwhelmed was such an inclusive and powerful way to describe how I was feeling, both when I was still working full-time and after I stepped back. The book describes us as "left-brained people." We are defined by the order and control that we have cultivated in our life to make our existence make sense. Sounds about right, eh? Post-concussion I was left in a situation where I lacked the ability to go-with-the-flow, so in response, I would act impulsively as a means of regaining control. My increase in impulsivity was directly related to my inability to make rational decisions in a timely manner the way that I could before the accident. I had a desire to pretend nothing was wrong and to be as concise or reactive to external stimuli as I had been before—this resulted in what appeared to be spontaneous and rash decision-making.

Dr. Denton also describes that pre-concussion, left-brained people are typically known for and identify with their organization, controlled thinking, and curated professional reputation.[44] We have created a "code of ethics" that forms our identity—what's right, what's wrong, very black and white. We, left-brained people, feel the need to find a level of control with the changes that are taking place physically and mentally. The black-and-white existence that left-brained people have carefully crafted is now shrouded in grey, and we feel ethically compromised and overwhelmed.

Understanding that I needed to let go of my need for controlling situations and narratives about myself went a long way towards forging a path that would support my recovery. I needed to find something that would support my ethical values and ingrained professional abilities, while integrating new strengths that I was discovering every day. This new outlook had a profound effect on my way forward after I quit work for medical reasons. I was dedicated to finding a new purpose.

I quit my doctorate after about eighteen months of trying to muddle through it after my accident, while still working full-time for most of that period. I was so disappointed in myself, but I had come to realize that not only was a doctorate very time-consuming, it was hanging over me like a cloud that was hindering my recovery. It wasn't the act of quitting my studies that was the most distressing part, I really just didn't want to disappoint anyone else. Quitting was embarrassing, an admission that I couldn't do it, I imagined my dad having a field day with my failure. More than anything though, I did not want to disappoint my doctorate advisor; he had always been there for me; He knew I was struggling, but he also knew that I needed to be the one to pull the plug. He couldn't tell me that I was incapable of completing the work. In the end, I knew it was time to hang up my hat and admit that my brain didn't function the way it needed for me to complete the required deliverables. It is possible to feel proud of yourself, ashamed of yourself, and worried about disappointing others all at the same time. It was the right decision though.

After quitting work and my doctorate, I had time to rediscover myself. I knew that I wouldn't be able to function in a military environment any longer. The first step was telling my primary care physician that my goal was no longer to reintegrate back into the military environment. I didn't think it was possible anyways, but my doctor was hopeful and entertained the notion until I told him that it was no longer my intention. This decision completely changed the trajectory of my recovery through the military. I was put on a path to medically release (retire), which included being posted to the Transition Centre. The Transition Centre is a unit that is specifically designed to work with ill and injured members of the Canadian Armed Forces. Whether your goal is to recover and reintegrate, or you are on the path towards medical release, all the services and support you need are located in one convenient location. I wish I had known about all the resources at the Transition Centre earlier, but again, being posted to that unit has a completely negative connotation in the military. The perception is that it's the unit where the sick, lame, and lazy go; and, it was the last stop, there was no coming back (complete garbage). I think that was the last straw. Once I realized exactly how many unfortunate, destructive, and discriminatory organizational biases that I had to overcome to get to where I needed to be in recovery, my distaste and distrust in the military institution was fused. I was done and ready to move onto a new future.

* * *

An appreciation for gardening was something that I inherited from my maternal grandmother (my nana) and my mom. We had this tiered, wooden, folding stand that sat in front of our living room window in the house where we grew up in Alberta. Every shelf was packed with different plants; watering was a chore that my sister and I used to fight over. My favorite plant when I was little was a spider plant (*Chlorophytum comosum*). I was fascinated by the way it self-propagated and made little babies that could easily be replanted. My nana was an African violet whisperer (African violets are from the genus *Saintpaulia*, and there are as many as twenty different species[45]). She had a wicker cupboard with drawers, overlaid with a clear plastic cover; it was overflowing with pots of fuzzy foliage with purple, pink, white, and almost blue flowers.

African violets are a complete mystery to me, I've never been able to figure out their requirements for survival. Nana had a knack for it though, and it was fascinating to watch her putter around the house, bottom-watering, and picking off dried leaves and spent flowers. When she died, my mom moved in with my poppa to help him out, and she maintained the African violets the best she could. Eventually, with subsequent moves to different residences, they've ended up with my sister. They are flourishing under her care, but they are truly family plants. A leaf propagation from one of the original African violet plants is coveted, and they've spread far and wide through friends and family.

While I was at RMC, we were allowed to have one plant in our room, if we chose, as part of our room inspection standard. My roommate and I went through many cacti and succulents, but nothing would survive in those old, dark, musty buildings. I didn't really connect with the fact that I was not choosing the right plants for that environment; something that was low light tolerant would have been more appropriate. Even then, whatever plant I would have chosen would have needed to be directly in the window to optimize the amount of light it would receive. There is no such thing as low light plants, only plants that can tolerate less light for a period of time.

My passion for plants, and ultimately their survival, developed out of necessity. I moved a lot over my career; my indoor plant collection was always a stabilizing factor in each new domicile. My urban jungle grounded me and made each new place feel like home, no matter how far I had moved. At this point in time, I definitely didn't consider myself a "plant collector." Yes, these people exist and I'm definitely one now, but at that time, I was only interested in greening up my space. I would buy a plant here and there from grocery stores and big box stores; I didn't know you could buy house plants in a nursery, I thought they were only for outdoor gardens. With my work schedule and other athletic and academic commitments, I didn't have time to plan and execute an outdoor garden.

Even if I wanted to do it at the time I experienced my concussion, my ability to garden outside was limited by the availability of space and the fact that it was the dead of winter in Ontario, Canada. I lived in a row house with my husband, my backyard was a postage stamp and all the landscaping was very low maintenance. There were a few small shrubs and the rest was mulched, covered in gravel, or with playground rubber mulch. There was absolutely no grass. It looked fantastic, but outdoor gardening was limited to container gardening. My obsession with indoor plants and collecting them happened inevitably—I had no outdoor space and it was freaking freezing!

Over the course of my recovery, I became an indoor plant fanatic. At first, I started my collecting quite naturally going to different local plant stores and nurseries. I wanted to try my hand at all the different *genera* of plants, and to figure out their care requirements. The different soil, watering, and light needs of different species fascinated me. I wanted to create environments where all of them could thrive.

Coincidentally, right when I was at the peak of my initial plant collecting surge, my husband and I decided to build a house outside the city. This presented an opportunity to design a space for myself within the house, where I could house my plants, focus on my new hobby, and figure out what comes next in terms of my future. We purchased a lot with twelve acres; the potential for development of the land to suit both Steve's and my needs was really exciting. Designing the house was an amazing experience! The build process was another story!

Our house was scheduled to be completed in the middle of November 2018. We sold our row house in Ottawa in October and moved in with my sister and her family, who had just moved to the National Capital Region (NCR). My plants were fielded out between my mother's, who had also moved to the NCR as soon as she found out my sister was going to be posted there, and my sister's houses. I literally took over their spare bedrooms with plants. Unfortunately, the closing date on our house kept being pushed back for varying reasons. I became obsessed with keeping track of what needed to be completed on the build and (basically) managed the project manager—who was unfortunately more hands-off than I wanted him to be. In reality, I had nothing else to do. I wasn't working and was living in someone else's house, continually focusing on my recovery was incredibly tedious. I was also starting to become very concerned about what I was going to do for money upon my impending release from the military. Intense worry about my future had started to take over again.

Due to the delays in our house closing, what was supposed to be a couple of weeks of couch surfing turned into four months. Many of my plants suffered over this time because I couldn't take care of both myself and my plants. Living in someone else's environment and trying not to be an inconvenience took a significant toll on my mental health. When we finally moved into our 75 percent finished new-build in February 2019, I was grateful for the space to expand personally and horticulturally. Interestingly enough, one of my new strengths was realized over the course of the house building process. As I spent more time with my plants, I became conscious of, and more sensitive to, recognizing "injustices," particularly when it came to inequality in relationships, for myself and for others. I pay more attention now to the people, their mannerisms, and to the tone of their voices. Because of this, I am more aware of when I'm being personally insulted or taken advantage of. Prior to my concussion, I would ignore or not notice when I was being taken for a ride, particularly at work. I just assumed that being overworked or overburdened was part of life, or part of my job. I have developed a sense of empathy for myself and others that correlates to a heightened reactivity in the face of perceived injustice. While I consider it an increase in my emotional intelligence, it is also a disadvantage because I'm more easily aggravated when I feel like I'm being mistreated. It is mind-boggling to me how I managed to put up with so much in my pre-concussion existence. As a result of my newly found courage in the face of injustice, I would barter, dispute, and debate with our builders to ensure that we got exactly what we paid for. That experience made me realize that I'm still intelligent and can get what I want, but now I'm not just relying on academics and process. I'm intelligent in a much more emotionally conscious and practical way; I learned to adjust to uncertainty and fight for what I believed was right. I had evolved.

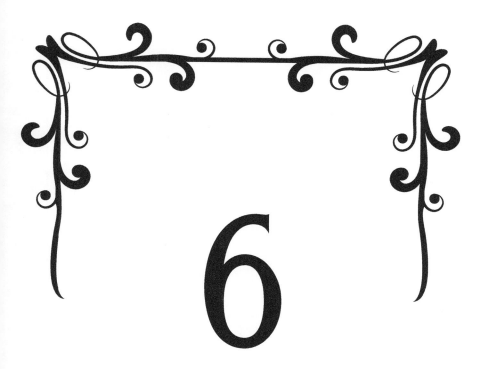

6

Stella Luna

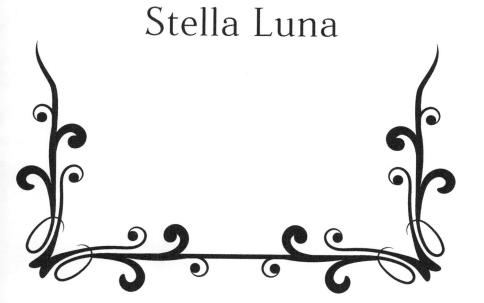

I met a very influential person in my plant care journey in January 2018. I met Velta at a concussion recovery yoga program called Love Your Brain.[46] Love Your Brain is a not-for-profit that was started by Kevin Pearce and his family. Kevin Pearce is a former US professional snowboarder who suffered a traumatic brain injury while training for the 2010 Winter Olympics. His recovery is documented in the film *Crash Reel*. Love Your Brain believes that yoga can be a powerful tool in recovery from post-traumatic brain injury. Velta had suffered a concussion while riding her bike. Oddly enough, we clicked immediately in class; I say oddly because I really wasn't connecting with anyone at that point. I was going through the motions of being nice and civil, but I was really struggling to connect with old friends, family, and strangers. But there was something about this stranger.

Both Velta and I were pretty committed to the Love Your Brain program and wanted to do as many of the movements as realistically possible within our ability. Looking back, I think the two of us were probably the best off, health-wise, in the class as well. Neither of us really identified as our disability, it was just the result of something bad that had happened to us. We could relate to each other and it wasn't just about our injuries. Velta and I are roughly the same age (I'm a few years older), and we were both in the same sort of place in our lives with respect to our significant others and careers when our accidents happened. I also found out later that her boyfriend (now husband) was also in the military. It was kismet really, like we were drawn to each other. Velta and I are completely different people though. She is a bundle of positivity and makes the best out of every possible situation. Her energy is boundless and she's one of the most selfless people I've ever met. I have learned a lot from her. When we met, I was in a dark place and was quite pessimistic, but I was incredibly motivated to recover to my pre-concussion state. Velta's realism and positivity were life-changers for me.

One thing that particularly inspired me about Velta was, despite her disability, she was really motivated to start her own business embracing what she had come to love during the course of her recovery. Velta is the proud owner of TerraVelta, a "growing plant" business (her favorite pun) that aims to recycle and reuse household items as pots and plant holders. Her brand is all about making plants accessible for everyone, while being environmentally conscious. She was running plant care workshops during her spare time when she wasn't saving the planet at her day job at Ecology Ottawa. The only way that I can describe it is that she had her proverbial shit together. I was completely awestruck!

Velta and I shared a mutual love for plants; the difference was that she was doing something useful with her new-found hobby. Her story is so inspiring it is worthy of its own book! Velta and I, quite literally, bonded over plants. We joke now that I imposed my friendship on her; I had made a choice that we were going to be friends and I wasn't giving her a say in the matter. It was exactly what we both needed though. It all started because I wanted to see what her workshops were all about. I started by attending one of her air plant terrarium workshops. I had fun . . . in a social situation! It was shocking. After that, I dragged my husband to a succulent in a beer can workshop—he wasn't overly impressed until he found out that he got to select and drink both of our beers before we could plant our succulents. Secretly, I just wanted to spend more time with Velta, supporting her business, without seeming too creepy. After that, I think she was endeared to me and I started working for TerraVelta at craft shows and fairs. I didn't work for money—I worked for plants. She was helping me get back into the world in a way where I was still in control. I could talk to anyone for an exorbitant amount of time if we were talking about plants; I could also step away from the booth for a few minutes if I was overwhelmed.

My friendship with Velta has changed my life and it has done a lot to steer me in the right direction, career-wise. In the summer of 2018, I was in a huge panic. I knew that I was medically unfit for the military, and it was only a matter of time until the paperwork was processed—I would be out on the streets, at least that's how it felt to me. Of course, the reality is that there is a process, which involves the military medical system assessing your needs and level of preparation for becoming a functional civilian. In total, this process took two years to invoke and my military release date will be July 21, 2020. At the time though, my brain was telling me it was time to panic and I needed to figure out what I wanted to do with my life.

All I knew up to that point was the military (I joined when I was seventeen), I was literally a product of the military institution. I had difficulty seeing what my transferable strengths were from military to civilian life. Yes, I was educated, and I had learned some project management, leadership, training, and research skills during this time, but could I now add some value to a civilian organization? Could I even be an engineer anymore? A project manager? Was my injury going to hold me back from being employable? There were more questions than there were answers because I had yet to be posted to the Transition Centre where people would help me recognize my worth. I felt like I had put myself in a box and that my experience was only useful to the Department of National Defence (DND). In reality, most veterans have difficulty recognizing that their worth is transferable to a post-military world. It is an issue that both the military and post-military service organizations are working to solve.

I began applying to every job that I could find on the Canadian Government job website and on LinkedIn that I was qualified for (even some that I wasn't) within Ottawa. I even applied to a job posting for director of the Science Museum! I definitely didn't get an invitation to interview for that one. It was all an act of desperation. I knew I didn't want to work for DND anymore, but I also thought that I wasn't ready to give up all the perks of a government job. I hadn't thought about my Canadian Armed Forces (CAF) pension or any veteran's affairs disability awards (basically a medical pension military people receive if they are injured during service) that

I would receive as a consequence of my twenty-two years of service. I was single-minded in trying to find a way to replace 100 percent of my major's pay check, and I was worried about having to settle for less. I kept applying to dozens of jobs even though I knew they would be inappropriate based on my struggling mental and physical health. I knew I would be putting myself back in the exact same position that I had been in when I was forced to step back from my job to focus on my recovery. My brain injury made me devalue my self-worth and everything that I'd earned prior to the concussion. Sure, I might not have been able to employ all of the skills or knowledge as adeptly as I had before, but they must still have been somewhere lurking in the corner of the depths of the abyss that was my brain?

The sad part is, just like my aversion to going to the doctor, my aversion to doing nothing (jobwise) was also a mindset that I had gained in the military. Malingering, laziness, and incompetence are faults. I couldn't see that what was happening to me was any different. My recovery and the time I needed to heal seemed to me like I was exercising those faults. I also didn't think that anyone else would see it any differently; even though if this was happening to one of my subordinates, I would have moved heaven and earth to make sure they had the time and space required to get better. In actual fact, the military gives you the time you need to recover, but it's a select few individuals, a few bad apples, who make you feel like you aren't doing enough. It is those bad apples who get under your skin, they make you doubt yourself; they make you feel guilty for trying to get better because, in their minds, they need you more than you need time to get well. Even though I had stepped back from my job in May 2018, my boss was still emailing me at my home address to get assistance with projects throughout that summer. It made me feel both mad and ashamed. Finally, by chance, the military medical system stepped in and they sent her an email reminding her that while I was on sick leave, I no longer worked for her. I haven't heard one word from her since.

In July 2018, I got an email notifying me that I had been chosen to participate in the first round of the selection process for a job in strategic planning with the Royal Canadian Mounted Police (RCMP). The job sounded super interesting. It was outside of my wheel-house, but again, my cumulative military experience and previous ability to think outside the box were seen as advantageous. The first round of the selection was an at home written exam; we were given two weeks to do it, and it was roughly four to five long answer questions. Doing the research for, and concocting the answers to the written exam was kind of fun. It was like playing make-believe with scenarios that had varying boundaries that you needed to work within, but a little imagination was valued. It allowed me to exercise my brain in a new way. I never actually thought my application would make it past that stage until I got a call from the RCMP Human Resources Department saying I'd been shortlisted, and that they wanted to start the administrative review process (criminal record check and confirmation of security clearance). Once that part was cleared, I would be through to the interview process. I standby the notion that participating in any interview is good practice, regardless if you get the job or not. So, I did. It was an interesting experience. I feel the nervousness that I felt before the interview was healthy. I left feeling like I had done a good job—like I had been able to hide my brain injury.

I went through the entire process from July to November 2018. I didn't even know if I was ready to get out of the military yet. All of my paperwork was still in limbo and I was in the process of being posted to the Transition Centre. I was creating my own perfect storm for a meltdown. If I got the job, I wouldn't know if I could say yes. If I did say yes, I'd basically be forfeiting the retraining opportunities that the military offers to its veterans who are being medically released. I wasn't processing the full weight of the decision; I was only worried about losing my job, a steady paycheck, and the creature comforts of government employment.

My sister, Carrie, is a personnel selection officer in the military; it is basically like human resources. We were still living with her at the time when she had helped me with my resumé, she had reviewed my take home exam, and she helped me prepare for the interview as well. Carrie knows me better than anyone else in the universe, but she's also more reserved and empathetic than I am. We joke that when I was born, I left all of my empathy in the womb for her and she got a double dose. Carrie doesn't speak her mind about people's personal choices unless she thinks it is affecting their health in a negative way. She was the one who kept reminding me that I'm still in the military, no decisions have been made yet with respect to my future, and that I had time if I wasn't ready to start a new job and expedite my way out of the military. She was there when I got the second call from the RCMP Human Resources Department telling me that I'm their first choice for the job, but that I need to go through a fingerprinting process and a deep dive through my background. I was flabbergasted that I had made it through. I was proud of myself, but I was also shrouded with doubt.

Carrie and I have a mutual friend that we met playing rugby at RMC, SueEllen. SueEllen is committed to the practice of brutal honesty, which is likely why she was one of the few people that I was still in regular contact with after graduation. With my sister just moving to the area, we all decided to get together at Stella Luna, a frozen yogurt shop in The Glebe neighborhood of Ottawa. SueEllen knew everything that was going on with me health-wise and career-wise. She was going through a similar career crisis, so she was easy to talk to about transitioning and shared expectations. It was October 11, 2018. I'll never forget that date because it was the day that SueEllen and my sister intervened.

If you've ever watched the A&E show, *Intervention*, you'll understand how being called out in public can be emotionally fraught and infuriating. Both SueEllen and my sister expressed their concerns about how hard I was pushing myself to find a civilian job. They pointed out the fact that I was missing an opportunity to do something I loved with my plants; I also wasn't giving myself time to recover physically or mentally. While I wasn't shocked that SueEllen had such strong opinions on my recent choices, I was surprised that Carrie was holding her ground. Both of them spoke and I listened in misplaced rage and embarrassment. My frustration peaked and I started to cry . . . in public. That was the tipping point. I knew what they were saying made sense, but I also knew that going out on my own, away from the comfort of a government job was really scary and overwhelming. Somewhere deep down I knew that I would regret it if I took the RCMP job. It just took two people bombarding me in public to shock me into realizing that I didn't want to work an office job again or have a boss.

SueEllen, being the loving and pushy friend that she is, signed the both of us up for a one-day entrepreneurship workshop. These workshops are run across the country by a registered not-for-profit, separate from the military institution, called the Prince's Trust. This organization was set up by His Right Honourable, Prince Charles, The Prince of Wales. One of the key areas this charity focuses on is providing entrepreneurship training to veterans and transitioning Canadian Armed Forces members.[47] I didn't know it at the time, but the prince's trust was going to inspire me to go out on my own, to build a business based on my love of indoor gardening, and to take the time I need to recover from my injury.

This workshop went through a series of speakers over the course of eight hours who spoke about the benefits of entrepreneurship, the basic steps you need to take in the province of Ontario to get started, and several validation exercises to help us refine our ideas for our potential businesses. The room was filled with soldiers and veterans from all different trades and with varying backgrounds. Listening to their motivations, ideas, and enthusiasm was really encouraging. We also learned that this one-day workshop could be just the beginning of our learning opportunity with the prince's trust organization; there was also a five day workshop that we could apply for, as well as mentorship opportunities. I was all in! I knew exactly what I wanted to do by the end of the day; I was going to open an e-commerce business selling rare and uncommon house plants. I had been a customer to the few businesses that existed in Canada that were similar, so I knew there was a market for it. Also, I knew that this business idea would satisfy my desire to be useful to society, while still allowing me to be me. I could continue collecting rare plants, I would get the thrill of the hunt sourcing my stock, and I could fulfill the plant dreams of other Canadians.

As I was driving away from the workshop, my head was full of all the perks of running my own business: I could make my own hours, I could choose the direction of the business, the type of stock and the prices, I would market the way that I wanted to, and would create my brand based on my values. As all of this was floating around in my head, the phone rang over the speakers in my car. It was the RCMP Human Resources Department. The strategic planning manager job was all mine, I just needed to let them know when I could start. I don't even know what I was thinking when I blurted out, "thank you, but no thank you!" except that I knew I didn't want the job, at all. I didn't even ask to think it over or to talk to my husband. I just said no. I hadn't even told Steve how awesome my day had gone. I just said no. It was so incredibly freeing! I did feel bad about leaving the RCMP hanging, but I knew they had a second viable candidate. I didn't go through the entire selection process thinking that I wasn't going to take the job; it was a month-long thought process, inspired by a combination of my friends, SueEllen and Velta, my sister, my husband, and the Prince's Trust that gave me the motivation and confidence that I needed to see the light. A collective effort for sure, but sometimes it takes a village to get through the shell of the toughest nuts.

That night I went home and registered my new business online. I even designed business cards through Vistaprint and had them mailed to my sister's house. I bought the rights to both the .ca and .com domains within the world wide web! I was committed. This was what I was doing and there was no changing my mind. I hadn't been so single-minded and driven to do something since before my concussion, or hell, even since trying to get into RMC! This was going to be my new future and I wasn't ever going to work for "The Man" again. Damn "The Man"!

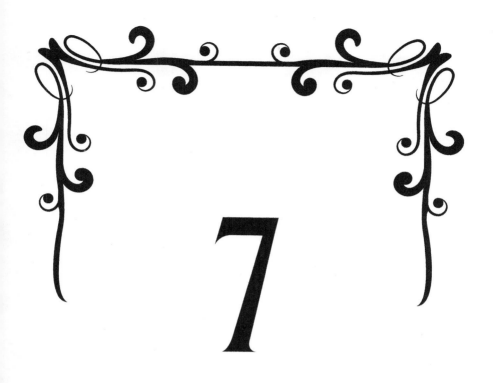

7

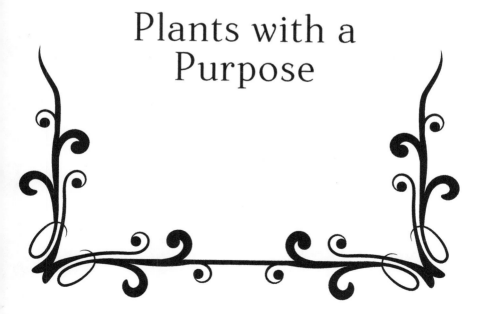

Plants with a
Purpose

Throughout my entire recovery process, my plants have been a central tenet of my self-care practice. I didn't realize it when I started, but the simple act of watering and tending to the needs of the plants was restorative for my mental health, my sense of purpose, and surprisingly, many of the physical skills that I'd lost, such as my hand-eye coordination and spatial orientation. The more time I spent focusing on my plants, the less time I spent pitying myself. They became a positive outlet for the negativity that had crept into my well-being.

As I got more and more interested in plants, I wanted to understand, without fail, why they made me feel better, why all I needed to do was enter the plant studio in our new house to feel emotionally lighter and more clear-headed. There had to be something to it. I wasn't the only one who had become obsessed with my indoor garden—it isn't called the "Millennial Plant Craze" for nothing. Our grandparents had African violet collections and sixty-year-old Hoya plants growing over the door frames in their houses for some reason. There had to be something about indoor gardening that is inherently good for our health.

I started looking into it a bit more and I discovered the book, *What A Plant Knows — A Field Guide to the Senses* by Daniel Chamovitz.[48] This isn't a book that preaches about the health benefits of specific plants. We all know that plants undergo photosynthesis, which uses light to transform carbon dioxide into oxygen, thus improving our air quality; we learn that in Grade two. This book essentially anthropomorphizes a plant's ability to sense and interact with its environment. Anthropomorphizing is an innate human tendency to attribute human characteristics and behaviors to non-human species or inanimate objects; we give our dogs or cats external monologues to try to explain their animalistic behaviors in human terms, so that we can feel more emotionally tied to them. It was interesting to understand how the results of simple experiments with plants, conducted by Charles Darwin and his son in the 1800s, could be used to help us understand how the species within the plant kingdom are aware of light and its directionality. The advent of genetic testing has allowed us to understand how plants have an awareness of their ever-changing "visual" environment around them. Plants have a sense similar to proprioception (something that I had been struggling with), which is why their roots always grow down into the soil and their stalks, foliage, and flowers are above ground. Plants even have a way of retaining information similar to our lowest level of memory called procedural memory, or the non-verbal way that we remember how to do certain things based on prompts from our environment.

If plants have all of these abilities: to "see," "smell," "feel," "hear," "know," and "understand" its orientation in space, then perhaps there are things that I can learn from them if I spend more time observing their habits, likes and dislikes, and daily routines. While not trying to sound too kooky, it was enlightening to know that plants had evolved and adapted ways to carry out these activities for which we rely on our "senses." I was struggling daily with my vision and hearing; reading Chamovitz's book made me realize that my thinking about seeing and hearing was very one-dimensional. Instead, I could improve my vision, and thus my sense of orientation in space, by relying on my sense of touch. I'm not talking about laying my hands on everything around me. I'm talking about observing things that I was feeling all the time but took for granted. Like the feeling of the sun on my skin as I get closer to a window, or a slight chill in the air when a door opens in another room. We feel all of these things every day, but we don't NOTICE them intentionally. This is where the mindfulness practice, as described in chapter one, became very helpful. By noticing more of the minor, nuanced things that happen when a person is speaking, such as their hand gestures and micro-expressions, I can better understand what they are saying even if my brain isn't processing the sound properly. I would have never been aware of these tiny changes I could make to the way that I perceive my cumulative environment, if I hadn't read *What A Plant Knows* or have integrated mindfulness into my daily self-care practice. Total life changers!

Okay, now that we've completely anthropomorphized plants, there is one myth that I would like to take the time to debunk. The origins of this particular urban legend can be traced back to the publication of two very culturally, popular books: *The Sound of Music and Plants* by Dorothy Retallack[49] and *The Secret Life of Plants* by Peter Tompkins and Christopher Bird.[50] Both of these tomes cite that talking or singing to your plants, and playing them certain types of music, will benefit their growth patterns. Now, if we are going to get technical, talking or singing to your plants is beneficial because you are supplying them with carbon dioxide, which they require to carry out photosynthesis, one of their requisites for survival. I would be negligent if I didn't point out that your plants cannot hear you, understand what you say, or sense different "vibes" from you or your recordings of Bach, Mozart, and Metallica. If talking to your plants helps you achieve a state of calm and reduced stress, then by all means, talk to your plants. While there has been anecdotal evidence that suggests that plants can "hear" by responding to sound waves of varying wavelengths and frequencies, they just have no need to listen to us. A recent study published in 2019 evidences that plants can sense the sound (i.e. the audio vibrations) of bees buzzing nearby, and they, in turn, upped the proportion of sugar in their nectar.[51] This research also suggests that plants can "tune out" unnecessary background noise, such as the wind. The study's authors note that this ability could improve a plant's potential to spread its pollen. These are evolutionary advantages that may help plants survive in the wild. There is no conclusive evidence to support that the sound of your voice, or the soft, soothing notes of Barry Manalo will change the growth pattern of your philodendron or make it "happy" so it sprites up after being under watered . . . Plants don't have feelings.

Before getting into a discussion about plants and their health benefits, let's first talk about the sudden resurgence in the popularity of houseplants within the millennial population. If we look at this demographic in a completely "by the numbers" sort of way, it is no secret that millennials are delaying the "classic" major life milestones (buying a house, getting married, having children, investing, etc.) because those things are just too damn expensive.[52] Very practical. The need for higher education to achieve a job with an adequate wage to meet these major life milestones has put many millennials in debt that they are struggling to repay. Lily Ewing, a Seattle-based therapist, believes that millennials are turning to plants as a way to fulfill their need for "connection and nurturing"[53] that they normally would obtain when they get married and have kids. Let's face it, plants are cheaper than kids, and sometimes, they are cheaper than husbands (kidding, not kidding)!

If a millennial did not have the privilege of growing up in a plant-friendly home, or their parents were part of the fake plant and carpet craze of the 1980s (my mom is guilty of both of these cardinal decorating sins), then they find their way to the houseplant world through social media. Instagram, Facebook, and YouTube are filled with visually pleasing accounts and channels for "plant influencers" (yes, it's a thing), plant collectors, and plant hobbyists. In the United States, the social media driven plant market has been responsible for millennials spending 25 percent of the record $47.8 BILLION dollars spent on lawn and garden retail sales in 2018.[54] Social media sets the trends for what the next "it" houseplant is, and thus, sets the retail value for these commodities. A plant that costs $25 at the grocery store in April, could cost $450 at a specialty store by the end of the summer.

Social media has also created easy access to an entire "Plant Community." There are real-life events to get involved in including: plant workshops, plant swaps, plant conferences, and the pinnacle of "plant culture," the International Aroid Society (IAS) annual show and sale (which moves around to different countries from year-to-year). The accessibility of the plant community, both in real-life and online, has encouraged millennials to flock together in solidarity for their plant fanaticism. In my experience, the plant community has been incredibly inspiring. It is low drama in comparison to other social media communities (we all remember the beauty YouTube drama between James Charles, Tati Westbrook, and Jeffree Star of May 2019). The plant community is supportive and kind; we help each other through mealybug infestations and poor lighting situations without judgement because we've all been there. I am appreciative of all the people I have met locally, in-person at community events, and online. The plant community is here to stay, and it's about more than social media street cred.

Aside from the sense of community and the fact that we can (erroneously) attribute human qualities to them, plants have been scientifically proven to be good for your health. If we extrapolate the scientific evidence to focus primarily on indoor gardens, the data tells us that these are the top seven reasons to maintain plants for your health:[55]

1. **Connecting with nature**—Natural environments that allow for the renewal of a person's ability to adapt to environmental stressors and offer physical, emotional, and mental wellness recuperation are called "restorative environments."[56] People have an innate need to connect with nature, oftentimes that isn't easy to do in highly urbanized environments. Environments where humans are encouraged to interact with nature, either organically or by design, have been found to mediate the destructive effects of stress by regulating mood and invoking a calming response. Restorative environments have also been found to increase cognitive performance through the reinvigoration of attention and focus.

2. **Increase oxygen levels**—Did you know that as urbanized humans, unless our occupation requires us to be outside, we spend upwards of 90 percent of our lives indoors? I didn't know until I started researching it. As it becomes closer to the norm to be jam-packed into office buildings, our health can become affected by the levels of carbon dioxide in our environment. Indoor plants, by virtue of their life processes, positively impact the levels of carbon dioxide in the air by replacing it with oxygen through the process of photosynthesis. By optimizing the plant's environment, ensuring adequate light and temperature conditions, we can improve a plant's

ability to increase the oxygen levels in our indoor environments.[57]

3. **Remove airborne toxins**—In addition to increasing oxygen levels, while simultaneously decreasing carbon dioxide levels, plants can also remove harmful chemicals that can build up in the air. We go about our lives surrounded by potentially harmful chemicals such as hydrocarbons, volatile organic compounds (VOCs), different ingredients in industrial cleaners, mold, particulate matter, etc. These can build up in the air, irritating your eyes, skin, and respiratory pathway. Many different houseplants are known for removing various types and levels of airborne contaminants; we call these plants "air scrubbers."[58]

4. **Medicinal uses**—In terms of directly using plants for medicinal purposes, there are thousands of documented cases of a particular plant having a medicinal use or uses. We used plants before we could commercially synthesize pharmaceuticals. Some examples of plants that can be grown indoors that can provide physical relief include: aloe vera to take the sting out of a sunburn, mint (*Mentha*) to calm gas and bloating, thyme (*Thymus vulgaris*) has antiseptic and antibacterial properties, parsley (*Petroselinum crispum*) can help cure urinary tract infections, etc. In a more indirect approach to considering plants as serving medicinal purposes, one study found

that bringing plants or flowers to a loved one in the hospital can actually improve their surgical outcomes.[59] The study authors found that patients recovered faster, tolerated pain better, and they required fewer pharmaceutical interventions for pain and inflammation if they had a plant in their room or a view of nature from their window.

5. **Promotes sleep**—This was a health benefit that I was particularly interested in, and I did quite a bit of personal research to find plants that I could grow, which would help my sleep patterns. First, simply increasing the oxygen levels in the room will assist with sleep (see point one). Next, I came across lavender and valerian, which are both easily grown potted indoors from seed. Valerian roots and leaves can be harvested and made into a tincture for use as a sleep aid.[60] The scent of lavender is known to have a calming effect, reducing blood pressure and lowering the heart rate, which will reduce your overall physical stress burden to help you sleep.[61]

6. **Improves mental and emotional health**— Indoor plants help reduce stress, anxiety, and depression. A study in 2015 presented results on how the interaction with indoor plants may reduce psychological and physiological stress by suppressing autonomic nervous system activity.[62] This means that your indoor garden can have a positive effect on your blood

pressure, heart rate, and the production of the stress hormone cortisol. Plants have an overall calming effect on our physical stress burden, which translates into a beneficial effect for our mental health because it changes how we feel and identify being stressed out. In the UK, doctors are prescribing houseplants to patients who suffer from anxiety, depression, and loneliness to lessen their symptoms.[63] Horticulture therapy is a recognized tool in the mental health treatment toolbox as it has been proven to help treat depression and anxiety, as well as treating patients who are dealing with trauma and dementia.

7. **Restoration of sense of purpose**—In 2007, in the UK, the "Gardening Leave" program was established as a horticulture therapy pilot project whose aim was to enhance the therapy experience for veterans with combat stress related mental health issues.[64] One of the primary outcomes of this study was that the participants felt a renewed sense of purpose, which manifested as an increased sense of pride, improved motivation and a sense of "giving back" as they were helping to develop the garden. The veteran participants began to look forward to their next plant therapy session. In my personal experience, this has been the greatest health benefit that I have achieved throughout my plant care journey.

Eventually, I hope to extend the mindfulness that I achieve through horticulture and my urban jungle throughout all activities in my life, whether they are intentional self-care activities or just day-to-day chores. Since taking up this urban jungle hobby and mindful horticulture, I have come closer to feeling whole again. I have realized the mental and physical benefits of staying in the present, not obsessively worrying about the future or regretting the decisions I've made in the past. The culmination of the scientifically-proven advantages and the less obvious application of mindfulness to horticulture has been instrumental in my recovery post-brain injury.

* * *

I will leave you with some activities to help you integrate plants into your life. *Appendix 3* contains a list of some plants and over-arching genera with their descriptions that are great for starting your urban jungles. Depending on how confident you are with your plant parenting skills, the list has been divided by "ease of care" ranking for your convenience. The ranking is based on my own personal experience, as well as through the absorption of knowledge from the plant community. I have also included a brief summary of how they may be specifically beneficial for your health in the plant descriptions. I fully encourage you to do your own research and understand the micro-environment within your own home in order to choose the best plants for your indoor house plant journey. *Appendix 4* is a list of some great websites, YouTube channels and "plantstagrams" (the term used to describe an Instagram account dedicated to plants) that you can follow. Come join the plant community!

Epilogue

Sweetlife Flora

The running joke in my family is that at least it's plants that I'm addicted to . . . there have been a few worse things that I've been obsessed with in the past, so I'm grateful that I'm now committing myself to healthier life habits. My plants and my implementation of a mindful horticulture practice have, quite literally, saved my life. I was in a bad place cognitively and emotionally during my first two years post-concussion; I struggled with the grief involved with recognizing the loss of my former self. I'm not the same person, but I'm now proud of whom I have become. I have passion again. I have a newfound appreciation for life. I am embracing my new talents and proficiencies.

Most of all, I am grateful for the support I have had through this recovery process. Meeting Velta was an incredibly serendipitous occurrence, I wouldn't be as emotional, or professionally complete without her. I am indebted to my sister, Carrie, and my friend, SueEllen, for their boldness and bravery in telling me that I was headed in the wrong direction and that they saw a hidden passion and potential within me. The rest of my family and a few friends, who I've managed to hold onto through this transformative experience, saw through the negative and to the core of who I was becoming, were fundamental in helping me accept the "new me." I am appreciative of the help that I received from my health-care practitioners. They took all of my concerns seriously, deservedly chastised me for not seeking help earlier, and they've collectively been with me throughout this entire rehabilitative period. I'm a work in progress, but they've stuck with me. I am specifically thankful for my primary health physician, Dr. Shane O'Neill, who agreed to continue being my family doctor after I'd left the military. This continuity in care will be instrumental in my ongoing recovery progress. Secretly, I know the truth, Dr. O'Neill likes that I'm a challenge! I keep him on his toes. Finally, I want to thank my husband, Steve. To say that I've been difficult is an understatement. His unconditional love, support, and commitment to our relationship has been inspiring. I couldn't have done it without him. He is my rock.

My life has meaning again. I look forward to the future. I officially opened my e-commerce business, Sweetlife Flora Inc., in June 2019. Sweetlife Flora sells rare and uncommon houseplants to the Canadian plant community. I enjoy working on researching, sourcing, and importing unique varieties of plant life. The process of acclimatizing these tropical plants to the North American indoor environment is satisfying and enlightening. I have learned so much in the last year as I've been setting up my virtual marketplace and have curated a revolving and responsive stock. Learning the sales and social media aspects of the business have been incredibly beneficial in satiating my ever-present desire for knowledge. I have also been able to use my platform within the plant community to raise money and awareness for some great causes including the Ottawa Food Bank and the Heroes Equine Learning Program.

The Prince's Trust has been an integral part of my success over the past year. I was accepted to participate in their five day workshop in Halifax, just two weeks prior to opening up my shop. This workshop, the speakers, and the student volunteers were super helpful in providing the exact advice and motivation I needed to kick me into high gear to put all the pieces in place before my opening day sales event through my Sweetlife Flora website. The Canadian Veteran's Marketplace on Facebook is a booming community—a venue for advertising veteran-owned businesses, allowing them to share their skills, talents, and wares with the public. There are several groups on Facebook and online (BuyVeteran.ca) that have been so supportive in helping me to promote Sweetlife Flora.

Being a veteran, I have accumulated all the skills I need through military service to be a successful entrepreneur. All the collective experiences over my career, including leading and advising soldiers, coaching, project management, teaching, research, conflict resolution, have culminated to make me the person that I am today. I needed people to remind me that my skills have merit outside the military environment. The Prince's Trust is doing amazing work to communicate the value of the skills and knowledge that Canadian Armed Forces veterans can bring to the Canadian economy.

I was also selected as one of The Prince's Trust alumni to promote their Buy Veteran campaign over Veteran's Week 2019 (Remembrance Day Week). The publicity that Sweetlife Flora received from this campaign was so incredibly overwhelming. I did interviews for radio and podcasts; my business was promoted on social media, and I was able to raise awareness about how to find businesses local to you and online that are owned by veterans and still serving CAF members. The whole experience was revitalizing. I felt like I was giving back and paying it forward to The Prince's Trust and the Canadian Veteran's Marketplace all at the same time. The Prince's Trust does more than just educate wannabe entrepreneurs, they inspire purpose. I hope to continue my involvement with this amazing organization in the future.

After my release in July 2020, I am going to take full advantage of the vocational rehabilitation program that is offered by the Canadian Armed Forces. In September 2020, I will be rejoining the land of academia at Algonquin College, taking their horticulture industries program. I am also currently enrolled in the only horticulture therapy course in Ontario that is accredited by the Canadian Horticulture Therapy Association. I want to be able to give back to the veteran, plant, and traumatic brain injury communities by learning how to facilitate and provide cooperative horticulture therapy practices under the Sweetlife Flora business umbrella. The Sweetlife Flora brand will evolve as I learn more and am able to incorporate this knowledge into different business lines.

Last, but not least, I want to build a state-of-the-art, sustainable, environmentally friendly and carbon neutral greenhouse on the Sweetlife Flora property. I want to learn how to expand Sweetlife Flora's current business plan into running a full-scale greenhouse operation for the propagation of tropical plants. This will allow me to streamline the Sweetlife Flora operation, and we will become less reliant on the importation of exotic plants. I also want to learn how to reduce Sweetlife Flora's cumulative carbon footprint by learning sustainable propagation and cultivation practices as well as by narrowing my market focus to primarily meet the needs of the plant community in my region. Establishing a brand that is representative of whom I have become and the service that I want to bring to the plant community has been incredibly fulfilling. I love being an entrepreneur and I can't wait to see what the future holds for Sweetlife Flora Inc.;

I have so many hopes and dreams for Sweetlife Flora. None of which would have been possible without the incorporation of a mindful horticulture self-care practice into my wellness regime. I have truly been propagated from the ashes of my former life.

Notes

Notes

Notes

Notes

Notes

Notes

Notes

Mindful Horticulture Planner

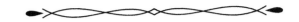

Week:

Sunday

Monday

Tuesday

Wednesday

Thursday

Friday

Saturday

Mindful Horticulture Journal

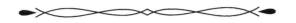

Date: Sunday

What observations did you make in your garden today?

What emotions did you experience
while caring for your garden?

What emotions did you let go of today?

Describe one thing, in your garden, you are grateful for.

Make some notes on your self-care goals for tomorrow.

Mindful Horticulture Journal

Date: Monday

What observations did you make in your garden today?

What emotions did you experience
while caring for your garden?

What emotions did you let go of today?

Describe one thing, in your garden, you are grateful for.

Make some notes on your self-care goals for tomorrow.

Mindful Horticulture Journal

Date: Tuesday

What observations did you make in your garden today?

What emotions did you experience
while caring for your garden?

What emotions did you let go of today?

Describe one thing, in your garden, you are grateful for.

Make some notes on your self-care goals for tomorrow.

Mindful Horticulture Journal

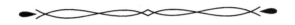

Date: Wednesday

What observations did you make in your garden today?

What emotions did you experience
while caring for your garden?

What emotions did you let go of today?

Describe one thing, in your garden, you are grateful for.

Make some notes on your self-care goals for tomorrow.

Mindful Horticulture Journal

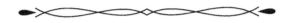

Date: Thursday

What observations did you make in your garden today?

What emotions did you experience
while caring for your garden?

What emotions did you let go of today?

Describe one thing, in your garden, you are grateful for.

Make some notes on your self-care goals for tomorrow.

Mindful Horticulture Journal

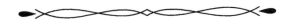

Date: Friday

What observations did you make in your garden today?

What emotions did you experience
while caring for your garden?

What emotions did you let go of today?

Describe one thing, in your garden, you are grateful for.

Make some notes on your self-care goals for tomorrow.

Mindful Horticulture Journal

Date: Saturday

What observations did you make in your garden today?

What emotions did you experience
while caring for your garden?

What emotions did you let go of today?

Describe one thing, in your garden, you are grateful for.

Make some notes on your self-care goals for tomorrow.

Appendix 3

Perfect Indoor Plants for Mindful Horticulture

The following table contains a list of some plants and general genus' with their descriptions that are great for starting your urban jungles.[65] Depending on how confident you are with your plant parenting skills, the list has been divided by "ease of care" ranking for your convenience. The ranking is based on my own personal experience, as well as through the absorption of knowledge from the plant community.

Google is your friend, look up each of these plants to see if their aesthetic appeals to you. Do research to understand the unique care requirements for each plant species. Know and understand the intricacies of your environment in order to better integrate and acclimate your plants into your home. This list is not exhaustive, there are thousands of species, hybrids, and cultivars that will do well indoors. Find the plant(s) that appeals to you.

Genus	Difficulty	Description
Sansevieria	Easy	**Scientific Name:** *Dracaena* is the over-arching genus for roughly 70 different species. The *Sansevieria trifasciata* is one of the most common houseplant varieties. **Common Names:** mother-in-law's tongue, devil's tongue, snake plant. **Description:** The *Sansevieria trifasciata* has spear-like foliage that is green and yellow/cream. **Care Instructions:** Tolerant of a wide range of light conditions; can adapt to a variety of indoor temperatures; water sparingly, once every two weeks in the summer and once a month in the winter. **Health Benefits:** Removes airborne toxins. **Pet-Friendly:** No.
Spider Plant	Easy	**Scientific Name:** Chlorophytum comosum. **Common Names:** spider plant, airplane plant, st. bernard's lily, spider ivy, ribbon plant. **Description:** Narrow green or striped green/white leaves with plant clones that grow on long shoots from the plant's center. **Care Instructions:** Tolerant of shade, but thrives in medium to bright light, keep the soil moist throughout the spring, summer, and fall. Allow the soil to dry between watering in the winter. **Health Benefits:** Removes airborne toxins, traps particulate matter in the air. **Pet-Friendly:** Yes.

Genus	Difficulty	Description
Aloe Vera	Easy	**Scientific Name:** Aloe vera. **Common Names:** Aloe. **Description:** Vertical fleshy foliage, the leaf fringes are ridged with dull barbs. The leaves are filled with a clear gel that can be extracted for use. **Care Instructions:** Bright or filtered light, water every two weeks throughout the spring, summer, and fall. Allow the soil to remain mostly dry throughout the winter. Avoid cold drafts. **Health Benefits:** Medicinal uses. **Pet-Friendly:** Yes.
Peace Lily	Easy	**Scientific Name:** Spathiphyllum is the overarching genus for more than 30 species. Spathiphyllum wallisii is the species most often found in stores. **Common Names:** peace lily, spath. **Description:** Dark green, lance-shaped leaves. Long-lasting white blooms. **Care Instructions:** Filtered sun or periodic shade, allow the soil to dry out between watering. The peace lily will let you know when it needs water—water when the leaves are very slightly wilted. Do not repot unless the roots have formed a solid mass and the soil is exhausted. **Health Benefits:** Removes airborne toxins and mold. **Pet-Friendly:** No.

Genus	Difficulty	Description
ZZ Plant	Easy	**Scientific Name:** Zamioculcas zamiifolia. **Common Names:** ZZ plant, zanzibar gem, zuzu plant, eternity plant **Description:** Evergreen aroid with an under-soil rhizome. Small oval leaves attached to thick stems. **Care Instructions:** Thrives on "neglect," adaptable to a wide range of light conditions, water sparingly in the growing months (when the top inch of soil is dried out), water once a month in the winter. **Health Benefits:** Removes airborne toxins, increases daytime oxygen levels. **Pet-Friendly:** No.
Echeveria	Easy	**Scientific Name:** Echeveria is the overarching genus consisting of approximately 150 species. **Description:** Huge amount of aesthetic variety. Compact succulent rosettes. **Care Instructions:** Bright sunlight, they will become etiolated if light conditions are inadequate. Drought-resistant, although prefer regular watering. Allow the soil to dry out during the growing season, echeverias will go dormant in the winter, minimal watering is required. A well-draining soil and pot are required. **Health Benefits:** Visually appealing, good plants for the work environment. **Pet-Friendly:** Yes.

Genus	Difficulty	Description
Cactus	Easy	**Scientific Name:** Inclusive of the plant family, Cactaceae, including 127 genera with approximately 1750 species. **Common Names:** Some of the more common cacti species have common names such as bunny ears, fishbone cactus, cowboy cactus, etc. **Description:** Huge amount of aesthetic variety. Generally evergreen, may or may not have sharp spines. **Care Instructions:** Bright sunlight, water moderately during the growing months, reduce watering to once a month during the winter dormancy period. A well-draining soil and pot are required. **Health Benefits:** Visually appealing, good plants for the work environment. **Pet-Friendly:** Yes, if consumed; No, if there are sharp spines.

Genus	Difficulty	Description
Pothos	Easy	**Scientific Name:** Pothos is the overarching genus consisting of approximately 55 species. **Common Names:** devil's ivy. **Description:** Fast-growing, robust vines with heart-shaped leaves. Leaves can be solid colored or mottled with varying amounts of yellow, cream or white. **Care Instructions:** Filtered bright or medium light, keep the soil moist throughout the spring, summer, and fall. Allow the soil to dry between watering in the winter. **Health Benefits:** Removes airborne toxins, increases daytime oxygen levels. **Pet-Friendly:** No.
Bamboo Palm	Easy	**Scientific Name:** Chamaedorea seifrizii. **Common Names:** bamboo palm. **Description:** Dense, lush green foliage that resembles bamboo. Long stems with arched fronds. **Care Instructions:** Low light conditions or shade are best, keep the soil moist, but not so wet the soil is water-logged. Avoid cold drafts. **Health Benefits:** Removes airborne toxins, increases environmental humidity. **Pet-Friendly:** Yes.

Genus	Difficulty	Description
Philodendron	Medium	**Scientific Name:** Philodendron is the overarching genus with almost 500 different species. **Common Names:** Some of the more common species of philodendron have common names such as elephant ear philodendron, heartleaf philodendron, selloum philodendron, etc. **Description:** Huge amount of aesthetic variety. May be a climbing or a ground-based self-heading species. In the wild, the leaves can be up to 2' in length and width. Indoors, 6-12" leaf length is normal, depending on the species. **Care Instructions:** Bright, indirect or filtered sunlight, water weekly and mist to increase the humidity around the foliage, wipe the leaves regularly to increase the ability for them to purify air. **Health Benefits:** Removes airborne toxins, increases daytime oxygen levels. **Pet-Friendly:** No.

Genus	Difficulty	Description
Monstera	Medium	**Scientific Name:** Monstera is the overarching genus with almost 50 different species. **Common Names:** Many species are collectively referred to as swiss cheese plants due to the leaf fenestrations. **Description:** Most monstera are green; there are variegated specimens (a genetic anomaly) that can have varying amounts of yellow, cream, or white. All species produce fenestrations within their foliage. **Care Instructions:** Filtered light, maintain moderate humidity by misting regularly, water only when the top of the potting mix is completely dry. Monstera produce aerial roots, a climbing apparatus (trellis or moss pole) will be required. **Health Benefits:** Improves mental and emotional health. **Pet-Friendly:** No.

Genus	Difficulty	Description
Aglaonema	Medium	**Scientific Name:** Aglaonema is the overarching genus for approximately 25 different species. **Common Names:** chinese evergreen. **Description:** Huge amount of aesthetic variety. Generally, have long oval leaves that grow from a central, thick stalk. Depending on the species, there are a wide variety of colors including green, red, pink, silver, white, cream, etc. **Care Instructions:** Low light conditions, keep the soil moist but not so wet the soil is water-logged. Avoid exposure to cold drafts. **Health Benefits:** Removes airborne toxins, increases daytime oxygen levels. **Pet-Friendly:** No.
Hoya	Medium	**Scientific Name:** Hoya is the overarching genus for 200–300 different species. **Common Names:** wax plant, wax vine, wax flower. **Description:** Hoyas are evergreen, perennial creepers or vines. They are primarily grown for their unique, powerful smelling flowers of varying colors and sizes. **Care Instructions:** Bright, indirect light, keep the soil moist throughout the spring, summer, and fall. Allow the soil to dry between watering in the winter. **Health Benefits:** Stress reduction. **Pet-Friendly:** Yes.

Genus	Difficulty	Description
Thanksgiving Cactus	Medium	**Scientific Name:** Schlumbergera truncata. **Common Names:** There are other species in the "holiday cactus" in the Schlumbergera genus, but the Thanksgiving cactus is the most common. **Description:** Drooping foliage with repeated, flattened segments. Flowers develop at the foliage tips. **Care Instructions:** Indirect light, keep the soil evenly moist, do not overwater. **Health Benefits:** Removes airborne toxins, increases oxygen levels at night, improves sleep quality. **Pet-Friendly:** Yes.
Dieffenbachia	Medium	**Scientific Name:** Dieffenbachia is the over-arching genus with 135 different species. **Common Names:** dumb cane. **Description:** Large oblong leaves that extend from upright stems. Dieffenbachia foliage typically displays some form of variegation. **Care Instructions:** Indirect sunlight, particularly avoiding direct sunlight in the hot summer months, which will burn the leaves. Keep the soil moist throughout the spring, summer, and fall. Allow the top of the soil to dry between watering in the winter. **Health Benefits:** Removes airborne toxins, increases daytime oxygen levels. **Pet-Friendly:** No.

Genus	Difficulty	Description
Dwarf French Lavender	Medium	**Scientific Name:** Lavandula dentata. **Common Names:** lavender. **Description:** Perennial flowering plant. Pale purple flowers at the top of long spike stems, slightly fuzzy green leaves along the entire length of the stems. **Care Instructions:** Direct sunlight, keep the soil moist without overwatering. When the flowers die, move the plant outside to overwinter, bring it back inside when it starts to bloom. **Health Benefits:** Stress reduction, improves sleep quality. **Pet-Friendly:** Yes.
Valerian	Medium	**Scientific Name:** Valeriana officinalis. **Common Names:** valerian. **Description:** Perennial flowering plant. Clusters of pink/white flowers on top of stems with round, dark green leaves with pointed tips. The leaves are fuzzy on their undersides. Please note that valerian is considered an invasive species in New Brunswick. **Care Instructions:** Direct sunlight or grow lights when grown indoors. Water on a weekly schedule. **Health Benefits:** Stress reduction, improves sleep quality. **Pet-Friendly:** Yes.

Genus	Difficulty	Description
Ficus Elastica	Medium	**Scientific Name:** *Ficus elastica*. **Common Names:** rubber tree, rubber plant. **Description:** There are several varieties of this species, however the most common type has large, oval, dark green leaves that extend from woody branches. **Care Instructions:** Bright, indirect sunlight, keep the soil moist without overwatering. **Health Benefits:** Removes airborne toxins. **Pet-Friendly:** No.
Alocasia	Hard	**Scientific Name:** *Alocasia* is the overarching genus of 79 different species. **Common Names:** Some of the more common species of Alocasia have common names such as african mask, jewel alocasia, elephant ears, etc. **Description:** Broad leaves on top of slim stalks grown from tubers or rhizomes. Leaf shapes can vary from arrowheads to heart-shaped. Colorful, pronounced veins, which exhibit a variety of textures from thick, waxy, slick, and glossy. **Care Instructions:** Bright, indirect sunlight. Water loving plants that thrive in high humidity. Keep their growth medium moist. **Health Benefits:** Improves mental and emotional health. **Pet-Friendly:** No.

Genus	Difficulty	Description
Anthurium	Hard	**Scientific Name:** *Anthurium* is the overarching genus for over 1000 different species. The most common species is the *Anthurium andraeanum*. **Common Names:** flamingo lily, flamingo flower, laceleaf, tallflower. **Description:** Dark green, heart-shaped leaves with spike-shaped stalks with varying flower colors. **Care Instructions:** Bright, indirect sunlight, keep the soil moist without overwatering, mist daily to maintain environmental humidity around the foliage. **Health Benefits:** Removes airborne toxins, increases daytime oxygen levels. **Pet-Friendly:** No.

Genus	Difficulty	Description
Boston Fern	Hard	**Scientific Name:** *Nephrolepis exaltata* "Bostoniensis." **Common Names:** boston fern, sword fern. **Description:** Long, arched, green, brittle fronds with a distinct rib running down the center. **Care Instructions:** This is the simplest type of fern to care for because its humidity requirements are moderate. Indirect sunlight. Keep the soil moist throughout the spring, summer, and fall. Allow the top of the soil to dry between watering in the winter. **Health Benefits:** Removes airborne toxins, increases environmental humidity. **Pet-Friendly:** Yes.
Fiddle-Leaf Fig	Hard	**Scientific Name:** *Ficus lyrata.* **Common Names:** fiddle-leaf fig. **Description:** Shiny, green violin-shaped leaves with a woody central stalk. Dwarf and regular varieties are offered. **Care Instructions:** Bright light, high humidity (but don't directly mist the leaves). Allow the soil to dry out between watering. Very sensitive to overwatering and drafts, does not like to be moved around. Keep the leaves free of dust. **Health Benefits:** Removes airborne toxins. **Pet-Friendly:** No.

Genus	Difficulty	Description
Maranta	Hard	**Scientific Name:** *Maranta* is the overarching genus for 40-50 different species. **Common Names:** prayer plant. **Description:** Grown from rhizomes. This is a clumping genus with crowded, oval leaves along sheathed stalks. In most species, the leaves are flat during the day to maximize light intake, but fold up as it gets darker out (hence, prayer plant). The leaves can come in a variety of colors, primarily green with distinctive veining. **Care Instructions:** High humidity requirement. Filtered sunlight, no direct sunlight. Keep the soil moist throughout the spring, summer, and fall. Allow the very top crust of the soil to dry between watering in the winter. Group marantas and calatheas together to increase the environmental humidity around their foliage. **Health Benefits:** Improves mental and emotional health. **Pet-Friendly:** Yes.

Genus	Difficulty	Description
Calathea	Hard	**Scientific Name:** *Calathea* is the overarching genus of several dozen different species. **Common Names:** Some of the more common species of Calathea have names like pin-stripe calathea, furry feather, etc. **Description:** Their foliage is incredibly unique and different to each species. Varying colors and patterns are available in different hybrids and cultivars of this genus. Calathea grown indoors are rare to flower. **Care Instructions:** High humidity requirement. Prefers shade. Keep the soil moist throughout the spring, summer, and fall. Allow the very top crust of the soil to dry between watering in the winter. Group marantas and calatheas together to increase the environmental humidity around their foliage. **Health Benefits:** Improves mental and emotional health. **Pet-Friendly:** Yes.

Genus	Difficulty	Description
English Ivy	Hard	**Scientific Name:** *Hedera helix.* **Description:** Extremely fast growing, evergreen vine clings to walls and structures. **Care Instructions:** Bright indirect light or shade, keep the soil moist throughout the spring, summer, and fall. Allow the soil to dry between watering in the winter. Requires moderate and sustained humidity. **Health Benefits:** Removes airborne toxins, increases daytime oxygen levels. **Pet-Friendly:** No.
Phalaenopsis Orchids	Hard	**Scientific Name:** Phalaenopsis is an overarching genus for roughly 70 species. **Common Names:** moth orchid, grocery store orchid. **Description:** Large, green paddle shaped leaves at the base of 1-3 stems that bear large, distinct flowers of varying colors. **Care Instructions:** Bright, filtered light and moderate humidity are required. They are not grown in soil, but rather bark chips. The plant should be regularly moistened to keep the epiphytic roots damp, but don't allow it to sit in water. Don't be discouraged when the flower dies, it can bloom anytime during the year. Proper grooming techniques will encourage re-blooming. **Health Benefits:** Removes airborne toxins, increases daytime oxygen levels. **Pet-Friendly:** Yes.

Appendix 4

Plant Community Resources

How You Can Reach the Author

Website: www.sweetlifeflora.ca
Email: info@sweetlifeflora.ca
Facebook: @sweetlifeflora
Instagram: @sweetlifeflora

Canadian Plant YouTube Channels

1. Plants Pots & What-Nots.
    "Plants, Pots & What-Nots"
    YouTube, accessed April 16, 2020
    https://www.youtube.com/channel/
    UCy4dJ8CObx0JKWFVodUhJWA

    Instagram: @plantspotsnwhatnots

2. House Plant Journal. "House Plant Journal"
    YouTube, accessed April 16, 2020,
    https://www.youtube.com/channel/
    UCKwhPQkQ1FF1le0MO4UfRHg

    Instagram: @houseplantjournal
    Website: https://www.houseplantjournal.com
    Book: Cheng, Darryl. *The New Plant Parent:
                Develop Your Green Thumb and Care
                for Your House-Plant Family*, New York:
                Abrams, 2019.

American Plant YouTube Channels

1. Mick Mitty. "Mick Mitty Plant Adventures"
   YouTube, accessed April 16, 2020
   https://www.youtube.com/channel/
   UCOKiWlaRrCjJ8GrdnqoDzMw

   Instagram: @mickmitty

2. Harli G. "Plants & Lifestyle"
   YouTube, accessed April 16, 2020
   https://www.youtube.com/channel/
   UCPlDlUEtyrOwDXOpls36b3g

   Instagram: @harli_g_

3. Legends of Monstera. "Legends of Monstera"
   YouTube, accessed April 16, 2020
   https://www.youtube.com/channel/UC9aJO_
   vRdGGhB_o-c-Vfdzw

   Instagram: @legendsofmonstera

4. Planterina. "Planterina"
   YouTube, accessed April 16, 2020
   https://www.youtube.com/channel/
   UCUIdHDKQIy-vr-D7M6KuRUQ

   Instagram: @planterina
   Website: https://planterina.com

5.   Summer Rayne Oakes. "Plant One on Me"
     YouTube, accessed April 16, 2020
     https://www.youtube.com/user/
     summerrayneoakes

     Instagram: @homesteadbrooklyn
     Website: https://homesteadbrooklyn.com
     Book: Oakes, Summer Rayne. *How to Make
                  a Plant Love You: Cultivated Green
                  Space in Your Home and Heart*, New
                  York: Optimism Press, 2019.

International Plant YouTube Channels

1.   Kaylee Ellen. "Kaylee Ellen"
     YouTube, accessed April 16, 2020
     https://www.youtube.com/channel/
     UCWRyi0LgQqAs7_Zz09VZA-Q

     Instagram: @kayleeellenofficial
     Website: https://www.therareplantshop.co.uk

3.   Roos Jemeis. "Yoga and Plant with Roos"
     YouTube, accessed April 16, 2020
     https://www.youtube.com/user/roosjemeis

     Instagram: @plantwithroos

5.   Plant that Plant. "Plant that Plant"
     YouTube, accessed April 16, 2020
     https://www.youtube.com/channel/
     UC07pXkYx0HRrrbfEi7PngPw

     Instagram: @plantthatplant
     Website: https://plantthatplant.com

Appendix 4

Amazing Plantstagram Accounts (Instagram)

@terravelta

@helloplanty

@thegardeningqueen

@thehouseplantinsider

@hiltoncarter

@plantkween

@nsetropicals

@keepyourplantson_la

@craigmilran

@foreverplanty

@thepottedjungle

@plantloversonly

@talkplantytome_

@botanicalfiles

@abotanicaltheory

@botanicalsandbillie

@arcticgardener

@houseplantsquad

@urbanjungling

@crazyplantpeople

@theplantjunkie

@houseplantfairy

@houseplantclub

@hothouse.jungle

@greeniegarden

@apartmentbotanist

@folia_folia

@plant.jungle

@rootandstemtropicals

@plantlovinghome

@be_nice_or_leaf

@wet_my_plants

@plantattic

@pflanzenarzt

@planttrekker

Plant Podcasts

1. Matthew Jackson and Stephen Ehlers
    "Plant Daddy Podcast"
    accessed April 16, 2020
    www.plantdaddypodcast.com

    Instagram: @plantdaddypodcast

2. Kevin Espiritu
    "Epic Gardening – Daily Tips & Advice"
    accessed April 16, 2020
    https://www.epicgardening.com/podcast

    Instagram: @epicgardening

3. The Royal Horticultural Society.
    "The RHS Gardening Podcast"
    accessed April 16, 2020
    https://www.rhs.org.uk/about-the-rhs/
    publications/podcasts

    Instagram: @the_rhs

4. Jane Perrone
    "On the Ledge"
    accessed April 16, 2020
    https://www.janeperrone.com/on-the-ledge

    Instagram: @j.l.perrone

Informative Websites and Blogs

1. "Welcome to Ourhouseplants .com"
   Ourhouseplants.com
   accessed April 16, 2020

   URL: https://www.ourhouseplants.com
   Instagram: @_houseplants

2. "Welcome to The Houseplant & Urban Jungle Blog"
   Invincible Houseplants
   accessed April 16, 2020

   URL: https://invinciblehouseplants.com
   Instagram: @invincible.house.plants

3. "For the Love of House Plants"
   The House Plants Expert
   accessed April 16, 2020

   URL: https://www.houseplantsexpert.com

4. "The Houseplant Guru: We All Need a Little Green in our Lives"
   The Houseplant Guru
   accessed April 16, 2020

   URL: https://thehouseplantguru.com
   Instagram: @houseplantguru
   Books: Steinkopf, Lisa E. *Houseplants: The Complete Guide to Choosing, Growing, and Caring for Indoor Plants*, Beverly, MA: Cool Springs Press, 2017.

Steinkopf, Lisa E. *Grow in the Dark: How to Choose and Care for Low-Light Houseplants*, Beverly, MA: Cool Springs Press, 2019.

5. "Your Complete Houseplant Care Destination!"
    Ohio Tropics (Raffaele Di Lallo)
    accessed April 16, 2020

    URL: https://www.ohiotropics.com
    Instagram: @ohiotropics

6. AboutSucculents
    accessed April 16, 2020

    URL: https://www.aboutsucculents.com

7. "Urban Jungle Bloggers: A Global Tribe of Plant Lovers"
    Urban Jungle Bloggers
    accessed April 16, 2020

    URL: https://www.urbanjunglebloggers.com
    Instagram: @urbanjungleblog
    Books: Josifovic, Igor, and Judith de Graaff. *Plant Tribe: Living Happily Ever After With Plants*, New York: Abrams Books, 2020.

                Josifovic, Igor, and Judith de Graaff. *Urban Jungle: Living and Styling With Plants*, Munich: Callwey Verlag, 2016.

8.   "The Plant Utopia: Exotic, Exciting, and
     Beautiful House Plants"
     The Plant Utopia
     accessed April 16, 2020

     URL: https://theplantutopia.com
     Instagram: @plant_utopia

9.   "Welcome to the International Aroid Society"
     International Aroid Society, Inc.
     accessed April 16, 2020

     URL: http://www.aroid.org
     Instagram: @internationalaroidsociety

Endnotes

1   Hanh, Thich Nhat. *The Miracle of Mindfulness: An Introduction to the Practice of Meditation*, trans. Hoe, Mobi. Boston: Beacon Press, 1976.

2   Brantley, Jeffrey. *Calming your Anxious Mind: How Mindfulness and Compassion Can Free You from Anxiety, Fear and Panic.* Oakland: New Harbinger Publications, 2007.

3   Harris, Dan. *10% Happier: How I Tamed the Voice In My Head, Reduced Stress Without Losing My Edge, and Found Self-help That Actually Works–A True Story.* New York: HarperCollins, 2014.

4   Michael, Raphailia. "What Self-care is – and What it Isn't," *PsychCentral (blog).* July 8, 2018. https://psychcentral.com/blog/what-self-care-is-and-what-it-isnt-2/, accessed February 21, 2020.

5   Hewson, Mitchell L. *Horticulture as Therapy: A Practical Guide to Using Horticulture as a Therapeutic Tool.* Guelph: self-published, 2004; Wang, Donna, and Thalia MacMillan. "The Benefits of Gardening for Older Adults: A Systematic Review of the Literature," *Activities, Adaptation & Aging*, 37, no.2 (2013): 153-181, http://doi.org/10.1080/01924788.2013.784942.

6   Guerriero, Rejean M., Christopher C. Giza, and Alexander Rotenberg. "Glutamate and GABA imbalance following traumatic brain injury," *Curr Neurol Neurosci Rep.* 15, no. 5 (2015): 27, http://doi.org/10.1007/s11910-015-0545-1.

7   Epps, C.T., and M.D. Allen. "Neurovascular Coupling: A Unifying Theory for Post-Concussion Syndrome Treatment and Functional Neuroimaging," *J Neurol Neurophysiol* 8, no. 6 (2017): http://doi.org/10.4172/2155-9562.1000454.

8   Epps et. al., "Neurovascular Coupling: A Unifying Theory for Post-Concussion Syndrome Treatment," . . .

9   "International statistical classification of diseases and related health problems." *WHO Library Cataloguing* 2010, vol. 2, 10th revision, pp 63-64, https://www.who.int/classifications/icd/ICD10Volume2_en_2010.pdf.

Endnotes

10   Kenzie, Erin S., Elle L. Parks, Erin D. Bigler, Miranda M. Lim, James C. Chesnutt, and Wayne Wakeland. "Concussion as a Multi-Scale Complex System: An Interdisciplinary Synthesis of Current Knowledge." *Frontiers in Neurology*, vol. 8. (2017): 513. https://doi.org/10.3389/fneur.2017.00513.

11   Simma, Burkhard, Jurg Lutschg, and James M. Callahan. "Mild Head Injury in Pediatrics: Algorithms for Management in the ED and in Young Athletes," *American Journal of Emergency Medicine* 31, no. 7 (2013): 1133–1138, https://doi.org/10.1016/j.ajem.2013.04.007.

12   Banks, Sarah J. "Chronic Traumatic Encephalopathy (CTE)," *Neuro-Geriatrics*, (2017): 183-94, https://doi.org/10.1007/978-3-319-56484-5_13.

13   Hay, Jennifer, Victoria E. Johnson, Douglas H. Smith, and William Stewart. "Chronic Traumatic Encephalopathy: The Neuropathological Legacy of Traumatic Brain Injury," *Annual Review of Pathology: Mechanisms of Disease* 11, no. 1 (2016): 21-45, https://doi.org/10.1146/annurev-pathol-012615-044116.

14   Maiese, Kenneth. *The Merck Manual Home Health Handbook.* Hoboken: Wiley, 2008.

15   Gouttebarge, Vincent, Haruhito Aoki, Michael Lambert, William Stewart, and Gino Kerkhoffs. "A History of Concussions is Associated with Symptoms of Common Mental Disorders in Former Male Professional Athletes Across a Range of Sports," *The Physician and Sports Medicine* 45, no. 4 (2017): 443-449, http://doi.org/10.1080/00913847.2017.1376572.

16   "Concussion in Sports." Government of Canada. Data reported from the CAN National Ambulatory Care Reporting System (NACRS), last modified June 2018, https://www.canada.ca/en/public-health/services/diseases/concussion-sign-symptoms/concussion-sport-infographic.html.

17   "Concussion in Sports." Government of Canada, . . .

18   Nguyen, Rita, Kirsten M. Fiest, Jane McChesney, Churl-su Kwon, Nathalie Jette, Alexandra D. Frolkis, Callie Atta, Sarah Mah, Harinder Dhaliwal, Aylin Reid, Tamara Pringsheim, Jonathan Dykeman, and Clare Gallagher. "The International Incidence of Traumatic Brain Injury: A Systematic Review and Meta-Analysis," *Canadian Journal of Neurological Sciences / Journal Canadien Des Sciences Neurologiques* 43, no. 6 (2016): 774-785, http://doi.org/10.1017/cjn.2016.290.

19   "TBI Get the Facts." Centers for Disease Control & Prevention, last reviewed March 2019, https://www.cdc.gov/traumaticbraininjury/get_the_facts.html, accessed February 22, 2020; Dick, R.W. "Is There a Gender Difference in Concussion Incidence and Outcomes?" *Br J Sports Med.* 43 (2009): i46–i50, http://dx.doi.org/10.1136/bjsm.2009.058172.

20   Covassin, Tracey, R.J. Elbin, William Harris, Tonya Parker, and Anthony Kontos. "The Role of Age and Sex in Symptoms, Neurocognitive Performance, and Postural Stability in Athletes After Concussion," *The American Journal of Sports Medicine* 40, no. 6 (2012): 1303-1312, http://doi.org/10.1177/0363546512444554.

21   Reed, T. Edward, Philip A. Vernon, and Andrew M. Johnson. "Sex Difference in Brain Nerve Conduction Velocity in Normal Humans," *Neuropsychologia* 42, no. 12 (2004): 1709-1714. https://doi.org/10.1016/j.neuropsychologia.2004.02.016.

22   Dick, "Is There a Gender Difference in Concussion Incidence and Outcomes?" i46–i50.

23   Covassin, Tracey, Swanik, C. Buz and Michael L. Sachs. "Sex Differences and the Incidence of Concussions Among Collegiate Athletes." *J Athl Train.* (2003): 38(3): 238–244.

24   Tierney, Ryan T., Michael R. Sitler, C. Buz, Kathleen A. Swanik, Michael Higgins, and Joseph Torg. "Gender Differences in Head–Neck Segment Dynamic Stabilization during Head Acceleration," *Medicine & Science in Sports & Exercise* 37, no. 2 (2015): 272-279.

25   Wunderle, Kathryn, Kathleen M. Hoeger, Erin Wasserman, and Jeffrey J. Bazarian. "Menstrual Phase as Predictor of Outcome After Mild Traumatic Brain Injury in Women," *The Journal of Head Trauma Rehabilitation* 29, no. 5 (2014): E1-8.

26   Ali, Siti A., Tahamina Begum, and Faruque Reza. "Hormonal Influences on Cognitive Function," *Malays J Med Sci.* 25, no. 4 (2018): 31–41, http://doi.org/10.21315/mjms2018.25.4.3.

27   Wunderle et. al., "Menstrual Phase as Predictor," . . .

28   Colantonio, Angela, Wanna Mar, Michael Escobar, Karen Yoshida, Diana Velikonja, Sandro Rizoli, Michael Cusimano, and Nora Cullen. "Women's Health Outcomes After Traumatic Brain Injury," *Journal of Women's Health* 19, no. 6 (2010): 1109-1116.

29   Ripley, David L., Cindy Harrison-Felix, Melissa Sendroy-Terrill, Christopher P. Cusick, Amy Dannels-McClure, and Clare Morey. "The Impact of Female Reproductive Function on Outcomes After Traumatic Brain Injury," *Arch Phys Med Rehabil.* 89, no. 6 (2008): 1090–1096.

30 Desai, Natasha, Douglas J. Wiebe, Daniel J. Corwin, Julia E. Lockyer, and Matthew F. Grady. "Factors Affecting Recovery Trajectories in Pediatric Female Concussion," *Clin J Sports Med.* 29, no. 5 (Sep 2019): 361-367. http://doi.org/10.1097/JSM.0000000000000646.

31 Colantonio, Angela. "Sex, Gender, and Traumatic Brain Injury: A Commentary." *Archives of Physical Medicine and Rehabilitation* 97, no. 2 (2016): S1 - S4; Cantu, Robert C., and Johna K. Register-Mihalik. "Considerations for Return-to-Play and Retirement Decisions After Concussion," *PM&R* 3, no. 10 (2011): S440-S444.

32 Breck, John, Adam Bohr, Sourav Poddar, Matthew B. McQueen, and Tracy Casault. "Characteristics and Incidence of Concussion Among a US Collegiate Undergraduate Population," *JAMA Network Open* 2, no. 12 (2019). http://doi.org/10.1001/jamanetworkopen.2019.17626.

33 Robson, David. "Why Women Are More at Risk from Concussion," BBC Future, modified January 2020, accessed February 24, 2020, https://www.bbc.com/future/article/ 20200131-why-women-are-more-at-risk-from-concussion.

34 Chen, Esther H., Frances S. Shofer, Anthony J. Dean, Judd E. Hollander, William G. Baxt, Jennifer L. Robey, Keara L. Sease, and Angela M. Mills. "Gender Disparity in Analgesic Treatment of Emergency Department Patients with Acute Abdominal Pain," *Academic Emergency Medicine* 15 (2008): 414-418, http://doi.org/10.1111/j.1553-2712.2008.00100.x.

35 Mollayeva, Tatyana, Graziella El-Khechen-Richandi, and Angela Colantonio. "Sex & Gender Considerations in Concussion Research," *Concussion* 3, no. 1 (2018): CNC51, http://doi.org/10.2217/cnc-2017-0015.

36 Tuthill, Azim. "Proprioception," *Current Biology* 28, no. 5 (2018): R194–R203, http://doi.org/10.1016/j.cub.2018.01.064.

37 Duffau, Hugues. "Brain Plasticity and Reorganization Before, During, and After Glioma Resection," *Glioblastoma* (2006): 225–236, http://doi.org/10.1016/B978-0-323-47660-7.00018-5.

38 "The International Classification of Headache Disorders." The International Headache Society, accessed February 24, 2020, https:// ichd-3.org/11-headache-or-facial-pain-attributed-to-disorder-of-the-cranium-neck-eyes-ears-nose-sinuses-teeth-mouth-or-other-facial-or-cervical-structure/ 11-2-headache-attributed-to-disorder-of-the-neck/11-2-1-cervi-cogenic-headache/.

39   Palenhan, Percival H., Brian M. Kelly, and Joseph E. Hornyak. "Classifications and Complications of Traumatic Brain Injury," *Medscape*, updated March 2, 2020. https://emedicine.medscape.com/article/326643-overview.

40   Amunts, K., O. Kedo, M. Kindler, P. Pieperhoff, H. Mohlberg, N.J. Shah, U. Habel, F. Schneider, and K. Zilles. "Cytoarchitectonic Mapping of the Human Amygdala, Hippocampal Region and Entorhinal Cortex: Intersubject Variability and Probability Maps," *Anatomy and Embryology* 210, no. 5-6 (2005): 343- 52, http://doi.org/10.1007/s00429-005-0025-5.

41   "Executive Dysfunction," Headway the Brain Injury Association, accessed February 24, 2020, https://www.headway.org.uk/about-brain-injury/individuals/effects-of-brain-injury/executive-dysfunction/

42   Marier Deschenes, Pascale, Marie-Eve Lamontagne, Marie-Pierre Gagnon, and Jhon A. Moreno. "Talking About Sexuality in the Context of Rehabilitation Following Traumatic Brain Injury: An Integrative Review of Operational Aspects," *Sexuality and Disability* (2019): http://doi.org/10.1007/s11195-019-09576-5.

43   Denton, Gail L. *Brainlash – Maximize your Recovery from Mild Brain Injury.* New York: Demos Medical Publishing, 2008.

44   Denton, *Brainlash – Maximize your Recovery from Mild Brain Injury.*

45   MacDonald, Elvin. *The World Book of House Plants.* New York: Literary Licensing, LLC, 2012.

46   "Turn Boldly Inward," Love Your Brain Foundation, accessed February 13, 2020 , https://www.loveyourbrain.com.

47   "Transforming Lives and Building Sustainable Communities," The Prince's Trust Canada, accessed February 14, 2020, https://www.princestrust.ca.

48   Chamovitz, Daniel. *What a Plant Knows – A Field Guide to the Senses.* New York: Scientific American / Farrar, Straus and Giroux, 2012.

49   Retallack, Dorothy. *The Sound of Music and Plants.* Los Angeles: Devorss & Co., 1973.

50   Tompkins, Peter, and Christopher Bird. *The Secret Life of Plants – A Fascinating Account of the Physical, Emotional, and Spiritual Relations Between Plants and Man.* New York: Harper Perennial, 1973.

51   Veits, Marine, Itzhak Khait, Uri Obolski, Eyal Zinger, Arjan Boonman, Aya Goldshtein, Kfir Saban, Rya Seltzer, Udi Ben-Dor, Paz

Estlein, Areej Kabat, Dor Peretz, Ittai Ratzersdorfer, Slava Krylov, Daniel Chamovitz, Yuval Sapir, Yossi Yovel, and Lilach Hadany. "Flowers Respond to Pollinator Sound Within Minutes by Increasing Nectar Sugar Concentration," *Ecol Lett*, 22 (2019): 1483-1492, http://doi.org/10.1111/ele.13331.

52   Bond, Casey. "Why Millennials Are Suddenly So Obsessed with Houseplants – It's much more than a social media fad." Huffington Post, last edited September 18, 2019, https://www.huffingtonpost.ca/entry/millennials-obsessed-houseplants-instagram_l_5d7a976de4b-01c1970c433b9.

53   Bond,   "Why   Millennials   Are   Suddenly   So   Obsessed   with Houseplants," . . .

54   "Garden Research: 2018 National Gardening Survey," The National Gardening Association, accessed February 20, 2020, https://gardenresearch.com/national-gardening-survey-2018-edition/.

55   Bringslimark, Tina, Terry Hartig, and Grete G. Patil. "The Psychological Benefits of Indoor Plants: A Critical Review of the Experimental Literature," *Journal of Environmental Psychology* 29, no. 4, 2009; van den Berg, A.E., and M.M.H.E van den Berg. "Health Benefits of Plants and Green Space: Establishing the Evidence Base," Acta Hortic. 1093 (2015): 19-30; Burchett, Margaret, Fraser Torpy, and Jane Tarran. "Greening the Great Indoors for Human Health and Wellbeing," *Final Report to Horticulture Australia Ltd*, 2010.

56   Berto, Rita. "The Role of Nature in Coping with Psycho-Physiological Stress: A Literature Review on Restorativeness." *Behav. Sci.* 4 (2014): 394-409.

57   Sevik, Hakan, Mehmet Çetin, Kerim Güney, and Nur Belkayalı. "The Influence of House Plants on Indoor CO_2." *Polish Journal of Environmental Studies* 26, 2017.

58   Luengas, Angela, Astrid Barona, Cecile Hort, Gorka Gallastagui, Vincent Platel, and Ana Elias. "A review of indoor air treatment technologies," *Rev Environ Sci Biotechnol* 14 (2015): 499–522, https://doi.org/10.1007/s11157-015-9363-9.

59   Park, Seong-Hyun, and Richard H. Mattson. "Ornamental Indoor Plants in Hospital Rooms Enhanced Health Outcomes of Patients Recovering from Surgery," *The Journal of Alternative and Complementary Medicine* 15, no. 9 (2009): http://doi.org/10.1089/acm.2009.0075.

Endnotes

60   VanZile, Jon. *Houseplants for a Healthy Home – 50 Indoor Plants to Help You Breathe Better, Sleep Better, and Feel Better All Year Round.* New York: Adams Media, 2018.

61   Bailey, Fran. *The Healing Power of Plants – The Hero Houseplants That Will Love You Back.* New York: Sterling Publishing Co., Inc., 2019.

62   Lee, Min-sun, Juyoung Lee, Bum-jin Park, and Yoshifumi Miyazaki. "Interaction with Indoor Plants May Reduce Psychological and Physiological Stress by Suppressing Autonomic Nervous System Activity in Young Adults: a randomized crossover study." *J Physiol Anthropol.* 34, no. 1 (2015): 21. http://doi.org/10.1186/s40101-015-0060-8.

63   Stillman, Jessica. "Doctors Are Now Prescribing House Plants for Anxiety and Depression," accessed March 21, 2020, https://www.inc.com/jessica-stillman/doctors-prescribing-house-plants-anxiety-depression.html.

64   Atkinson, Jacqueline. "An Evaluation of the Gardening Leave Project for Ex-Military Personnel with PTSD and Other Combat Related Mental Health Problems," accessed February 23, 2020, https://lx.iriss.org.uk/content/evaluation-gardening-leave-project-ex-military-personnel-ptsd-and-other-combat-related.

65   VanZile, *Houseplants for a Healthy Home.*

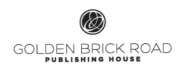

GOLDEN BRICK ROAD
PUBLISHING HOUSE

Link arms with us as we pave new paths to a better and more expansive world.

Golden Brick Road Publishing House (GBRPH) is a small, independently initiated boutique press created to provide social-innovation entrepreneurs, experts, and leaders a space in which they can develop their writing skills and content to reach existing audiences as well as new readers.

Serving an ambitious catalogue of books by individual authors, GBRPH also boasts a unique co-author program that capitalizes on the concept of "many hands make light work." GBRPH works with our authors as partners. Thanks to the value, originality, and fresh ideas we provide our readers, GBRPH books are now available in bookstores across North America.

We aim to develop content that effects positive social change while empowering and educating our members to help them strengthen themselves and the services they provide to their clients.

Iconoclastic, ambitious, and set to enable social innovation, GBRPH is helping our writers/partners make cultural change one book at a time.

Inquire today at www.goldenbrickroad.pub

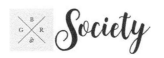